ESSENTIALS
OF FIRE SERVICE FIRST AID

Daniel Limmer • Michael Grill

Medical Editor
Edward T. Dickinson, M.D., NREMT-P, FACEP

IFSTA Senior Editor
Michael A. Wieder

Taken from

Fire Service First Responder
by Daniel Limmer, Michael Grill

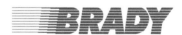

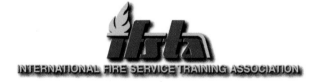

INTERNATIONAL FIRE SERVICE TRAINING ASSOCIATION

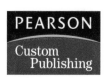

PEARSON
Custom Publishing

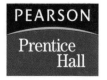

PEARSON
Prentice Hall

Cover design: Fire Protection Publications Design Staff

Taken from:

Fire Service First Responder
by Daniel Limmer and Michael Grill
Copyright © 2000 by Prentice-Hall, Inc.
A Pearson Education Company
Upper Saddle River, New Jersey 07458

This special edition published in cooperation with Pearson Custom Publishing.

Printed in the United States of America

10 9 8 7 6 5 4 3 2 1

ISBN 0-536-80610-1

BA 998890

JP

Please visit our web site at *www.pearsoncustom.com*

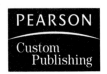
PEARSON CUSTOM PUBLISHING
75 Arlington Street, Suite 300, Boston, MA 02116
A Pearson Education Company

To Sarah Katherine, my Little Miss Magic—DL

Dennis Eaton, thanks for being a mentor, guide, and confidant.

Jeff Dyar, thanks for believing in me and giving me a chance years ago. My wife Sam and kids Moe and Lacey Ella, thanks for being patient and loving me. Behind every successful man is a supportive wife and a very surprised mother-in-law!—MG

Contents

Preface

At its inception, and for many years thereafter, the fire service had a single mission: protect the public from the ravages of fire. Over time the fire service began to assume other duties, including rescue services, hazardous materials response, and emergency medical services. In most communities, the fire department of today is truly a multi-disciplined service-providing agency.

Of these assumed roles, the provision of emergency medical services has perhaps had the largest impact on the fire service in terms of additional training, increased responses, and increased interaction with the public. Although a very few career fire departments still do not respond to medical emergencies, most career and many volunteer fire departments provide some level of emergency medical response to their communities. This response ranges from basic life support first responder service to full advanced life support ambulance service. Each community must determine their fire department's level of responsibility in the emergency medical system and then the training of the firefighters must be commensurate with that level of service.

Laws and standards for the minimum training of emergency responders who perform first aid duties for the pubic vary. Most jurisdictions require responders who treat the public to be trained at least to the level of a First Responder as defined in the U.S. DOT's First Responder National Curriculum. Today, many fire departments greatly exceed this minimum and require firefighters to be certified as emergency medical technicians (EMTs) or paramedics.

Because of the inherent dangers associated with the fire fighting profession, all firefighters, whether or not they personally or their departments are charged with providing medical service to the public, should have a basic level of first aid knowledge so that they may react properly if they or one of their fire fighting comrades are injured in the performance of their duties. For this reason, the National Fire Protection Association's (NFPA) committee on Fire Fighter Professional Qualifications (NFPA 1001) included the following requirement in their 2002 edition:

4.3 Emergency Medical Care. Minimum emergency medical care performance capabilities for entry level personnel shall be developed and validated by the authority having jurisdiction to include infection control, CPR, bleeding control, and shock management.

A similar requirement appeared as Objective 2-3 in the 1997 version of NFPA 1001.

The Essentials of Fire Service First Aid contains information that allows firefighters to learn the minimum first aid requirements contained in NFPA 1001. The information contained in this document was adapted from ***Fire Service First Responder***, which was produced by Brady Publishing and validated by the International Fire Service Training Association. Fire departments that require firefighters to be certified first responders should use ***Fire Service First Responder*** or a similar manual and an appropriate curriculum to meet that level of certification and training.

Acknowledgments

PROGRAM DEVELOPMENT

We would like to thank IFSTA, our Medical Editor, and the many members of the Brady team for the skill and dedication they have brought to developing *Fire Service First Responder*. The Brady team works together with a strong sense of professionalism, one that we greatly admire.

IFSTA Validating Committee The process of creating this book involved an extensive review and validation process. The IFSTA validation team met three times. (Please see a list of their names on page x.) During our meetings, we shared ideas and laughs. It was a great process that involved some of the finest people the fire service has to offer. Thank you. Thanks also to Mike Wieder of IFSTA for his support and organization during the creation of this textbook.

Medical Editor Edward T. Dickinson, MD, NREMT-P FACEP, is Medical Editor for *Fire Service First Responder*. We are always grateful for the keen eye that Ed brings to his review of material. His advice and observations have helped us stay current in a time of rapidly changing medicine and new curricula. Ed's knowledge, street experience, and high standards (combined with the fact that he was an English major in college) have helped us tremendously. Ed's contributions to this text have been invaluable.

Brady/Prentice Hall Health *Fire Service First Responder* is the result of many talented people working together. We gratefully acknowledge the tireless effort and attention to detail Jo Cepeda, our editor, adds to this and every project she works on. Editors make authors look good, and we are glad to have Jo working with us. At Brady, Lois Berlowitz is an advocate, a taskmaster, and a true professional in every sense of the word. A day cannot go by without appreciating Jo and Lois and what they have done for this project.

Photos are an important part of every textbook. Photos provide instruction, feeling, and examples. A book full of great words still is not complete without great photographs. Michal Heron, Managing Photography Editor, works tirelessly to ensure accurate, quality photographs and a clean, refreshing look to the text. Thank you. Anyone who has ever worked a photo shoot with Michal can attest to her quest for perfection. We must also thank all who worked as models and technical advisors. Working on the photos in this text involved long, hot days in the sun (and sometimes in fully encapsulated suits). As authors, we appreciate the efforts of everyone who made the book look great.

The production crew for this text, including Pat Walsh, Julie Boddorf, and Ilene Sanford are usually acknowledged, but perhaps not enough. Writing a book is only one part of the process that brings this book to you. Assuring the book is printed, that the photos are in the right places, and that it looks as good as we envision rests largely on these people. And they do so well.

During the production of this textbook there were changes in publishers. We worked with Susan Katz, our friend and publisher, for many years. It was Susan's vision that brought this book and others about. Susan's way of "doing business" brought a style to publishing that is unique and certainly appreciated over the many years we have had the pleasure of working with her. Susan made the business of publishing an art form. She will be truly missed. We wish Susan happiness and success in the future. Carol Sobel, Susan's assistant, was a constant voice behind the scenes. We talked to and relied on Carol for many things over the years. Her helpfulness and kindness will never be forgotten.

Julie Alexander has the responsibility of taking over a job held by Susan. These were "big shoes to fill," and Julie has done well. We have enjoyed working with Julie as she begins what we are sure will be a long and productive stay at Brady. Julie's energy and ideas are strong, even contagious. We look forward to a long and positive relationship with our new publisher.

Our marketing and sales force must also be commended. Tiffany Price and Cindy Frederick are driven, creative, and appreciated. Judy Streger has worked both marketing and editorial functions during the creation of this book. Judy's input and friendship is always appreciated. Judy Stamm and the sales reps work to get our book out there, and we thank all of you.

Last, but certainly not least, we would like to acknowledge our friends and colleagues Brent Hafen and Keith Karren. Brent and Keith began in the book business long ago. Their efforts and vision in bringing First Responder books from their infancy to where they are today must be noted. We gratefully acknowledge the contributions made to this text and to the field of EMS.

IFSTA VALIDATING COMMITTEE

Acknowledgment and special thanks are extended to the members of the IFSTA validating committee who contributed their time, wisdom, and knowledge to a thorough review of the manuscript for this book.

IFSTA/Fire Protection Publications Staff Liaison
Michael A. Wieder
Fire Protection Publications
Oklahoma State University
Stillwater, OK

Mike Buscher
Omaha Fire Department
Omaha, NE

Stephen W. Carrier, Sr.
Riverbend Career & Technical Center
Bradford, VT

Gary Davis
Oklahoma City Fire Department
Oklahoma City, OK

Beverly Deister
Reno County EMS
Hutchinson, KS

Jerome Harvey
City of Lead Fire Department
Lead, SD

William J. Mackreth
Wasilla, AK

Mark Monroe
Reichhold Chemicals, Inc.
Valley Park, MO

Bill Roth
Hemet Fire Department
Hemet, CA

REVIEWERS

Our thanks to the many people involved in manuscript review for their feedback and suggestions.

Gary Ferrucci, EMT-CC PC
Nassau County Police Department
Mineola, NY

Capt. Krista Wyatt
Lebanon Fire Division
Lebanon, OH

Capt. William Seward, III
Director of Training
Department of Fire Service
City of New Haven, CT

Lonnie D. Inzer
Lieutenant—Colorado Springs Fire Department
Fire Science Coordinator—Pikes Peak
   Community College, CO

Michael Zanotti, CEM, NREMT-P
Baker Heights Fire Department, WV

Stanley C. Vinson
Fire Service Captain
Mobile Fire-Rescue Department, AL

Al Lewin, EMT-P/Instructor
Auburn Emergency Squad, IL

Deputy Chief Bill Madison
Lincoln Fire Department
Lincoln, NE

Bradley Golden, RN, EMT-P, AAEMT
Jackson Fire Rescue
Jackson, MO

Sean Wilson AEMT-I-CIC
EMS Program
Fulton Montgomery Community College
New York State Academy of Fire Science
   Adjunct-CIC, NY

David W. Akers, EMT-B
Coordinator/Instructor
Sierra Fire Academy
Tollhouse, CA

Stephen Bardwell
Mississippi State Fire Academy
Jackson, MS

Lynn Lybrook, EMT-P, EMS Field Training
   Coordinator
Alabama Fire College
Tuscaloosa, AL

Dennis Matty, Lieutenant
Miramar Fire Rescue, FL

Robert C. Hecker, Fire Captain, Paramedic
   Instructor
St. Tammany Parish Fire District #4, LA

Capt. Tony C. Watson, EMT-P
Instructor/Coordinator
Pigeon Forge Fire Department, TN

James B. Miller, EMT-P
EMS Coordinator
Fire and Emergency Services
Fort Sam Houston, TX

Capt. Steve Moffitt
EMS Division
Alabama Fire College
Tuscaloosa, AL

Mark Stewart
Louisiana State University Fire and Emergency
   Training Institute, LA

Chip Boehm, RN, EMT-P/FF
EMS Education/QI Officer
Portland Fire Department
Portland, ME

PHOTO ACKNOWLEDGMENTS

All photographs not credited adjacent to the photograph were photographed on assignment for Brady/Prentice Hall Health.

Organizations: We wish to thank the following organizations for their valuable assistance in creating the photo program for this edition:

American Medical Response, Hemet Valley
   Ambulance Service: Laurie Hunter, Director
   of Government Affairs; Jack Hansen,
   Operations Manager; Art Durbin, EMT-P,
   RN, BS, Clinical Manager

Fire Protection Publications, IFSTA: Michael A.
   Wieder

City of Hemet Fire Department, Hemet, CA:
   David A. Van Verst, Battalion Chief

Plano Fire and Rescue, Plano, Texas: Chief Bill
   Peterson; EMS Coordinator Ken Klein;
   Monique Cardwell, Public Education

Reichhold Chemicals, Inc., Newark, NJ:
   Ron Kurtz, Jack Connolly, EMS Technician
TACTRON Incident Control Products,
   Sherwood, Oregon

Technical Advisors: Our thanks to the following people for providing extraordinary assistance and valuable technical support during the photo shoots:

Art Durbin, EMT-P, RN, BS, Clinical Manager,
   Hemet Valley Ambulance Service,
   American Medical Response, Hemet, CA

Jack Connolly, EMS Technician,
   Reichhold Chemicals, Inc., Newark, NJ

Ken Klein, RN, EMT-P Coordinator, Kenneth
   C. Larsen EMTP-TACT, Plano Fire and
   Rescue, Plano, TX

Daniel Pohan, Savox Lifeline Communications,
   Ridgefield, NJ

Brian Rathbone, Hazmat/Rescue Training
   Consultant, The Mechanical Advantage,
   Hackettstown, NJ

Captain William C. Roth, and Jim Snodgrass,
   Battalion Chief, City of Hemet Fire
   Department, Hemet, CA

Happy Snodgrass, Officer, City of Hemet
   Police Department, Hemet, CA

Scene Safety and the Well-Being of the First Responder

CHAPTER
1

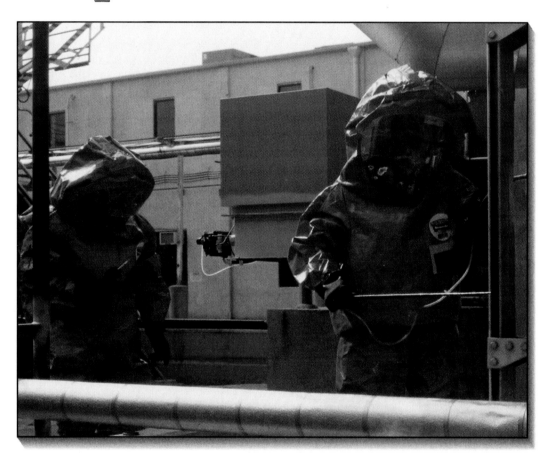

*I*NTRODUCTION   *As a fire service First Responder, your safety always comes first. It comes before the patient and before any bystander at the scene. The reason is simple. If you are injured, you lose the ability to help those who need you and, instead of providing emergency care, you end up needing it.*

Many elements make up rescuer safety. Most basic training programs teach how to react safely to a variety of environmental threats, such as fire and flood. But the most common threat to a rescuer is his or her attitude towards safety. This chapter outlines the basic steps you should take to maintain your well-being. It includes an introduction to scene safety, how to anticipate and handle the emotional aspects of emergencies, and how to protect yourself against infection.

OBJECTIVES

Cognitive, affective, and psychomotor objectives are from the U.S. DOT's "First Responder: National Standard Curriculum." Enrichment objectives, if any, identify supplemental material.

Cognitive

1-2.1 List possible emotional reactions that the First Responder may experience when faced with trauma, illness, death, and dying. (pp. 3–5)

1-2.2 Discuss the possible reactions that a family member may exhibit when confronted with death and dying. (pp. 6–8)

1-2.3 State the steps in the First Responder's approach to the family confronted with death and dying. (pp. 6–8)

1-2.4 State the possible reactions that the family of the First Responder may exhibit. (p. 5)

1-2.5 Recognize the signs and symptoms of critical incident stress. (pp. 3–4)

1-2.6 State possible steps that the First Responder may take to help reduce/alleviate stress. (pp. 4–5)

1-2.7 Explain the need to determine scene safety. (pp. 13–16)

1-2.8 Discuss the importance of body substance isolation (BSI). (pp. 8–13)

1-2.9 Describe the steps the First Responder should take for personal protection from airborne and bloodborne pathogens. (pp. 8–13)

1-2.10 List the personal protective equipment necessary for each of the following situations: (pp. 8–16)
  — Hazardous materials
  — Rescue operations
  — Violent scenes
  — Crime scenes
  — Electricity
  — Water and ice
  — Exposure to bloodborne pathogens
  — Exposure to airborne pathogens

Affective

1-2.11 Explain the importance of serving as an advocate for the use of appropriate protective equipment. (p. 12)

1-2.12 Explain the importance of understanding the response to death and dying and communicating effectively with the patient's family. (pp. 6–8)

1-2.13 Demonstrate a caring attitude towards any patient with illness or injury who requests emergency medical services. (p. 7–8)

1-2.14 Show compassion when caring for the physical and mental needs of patients. (pp. 6–8)

1-2.15 Participate willingly in the care of all patients. (p. 7)

1-2.16 Communicate with empathy to patients being cared for, as well as with family members, and friends of the patient. (pp. 6–8)

Psychomotor

1-2.17 Given a scenario with potential infectious exposure, the First Responder will use appropriate personal protective equipment. At the completion of the scenario, the First Responder will properly remove and discard the protective garments. (p. 12)

1-2.18 Given the above scenario, the First Responder will complete disinfection/cleaning and all reporting documentation. (pp. 11–13)

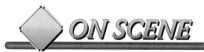

DISPATCH

My partner and I are First Responders with our volunteer fire department. We were finishing up our monthly training one Saturday and were just about to leave the station, when dispatch called. There was an assault with one person bleeding at 99 Snyder Drive.

We got in the rescue truck. It was my partner's turn to drive. I got out the town map and located the residence. On the way, I mentally went over the procedures for body substance isolation and bleeding control.

SCENE SIZE-UP

En route, we asked dispatch if the police were responding. She stated they were. About one block from the patient's house, we decided to stage our vehicle until the police could determine if the scene was safe to enter. After a few minutes, dispatch informed us that the police were on scene and were requesting our response.

Arriving at the address, we parked our vehicle behind the police squad cars. Exiting our vehicle, I immediately heard men yelling and glass breaking. Loud thumps and scuffling made it obvious that an altercation was occurring. It became clear to me and my partner that, although the police had requested our response, things were not quite under control yet.

Caution will help you to recognize potential dangers at an emergency scene. But is violence the only kind of danger you may face? Consider your answer as you read this chapter.

SECTION 1 EMOTIONAL ASPECTS OF EMERGENCY CARE

Stress is any change in the body's internal balance. It occurs when outside demands are greater than the body's resources. High-stress situations include multiple-casualty incidents, injury to an infant or child, death of a patient, an amputation, violence, abuse, and injury or death of a coworker.

A First Responder's initial response to stress may include weakness, nausea, vomiting, or fainting. You can help avoid these reactions by using the following techniques:

◆ Close your eyes and take several long, deep breaths. Focus on counting each breath. When you feel more in control, return to giving emergency care.

◆ Change your thought patterns. Silently hum a soothing tune to yourself, or visualize a happy outcome for the call.

◆ Eat properly to maintain your blood sugar. Low blood sugar can add to a fainting problem.

Stress Management

As a fire service First Responder, you will be exposed to a great deal of stress when meeting the needs of your patients. Some First Responders tend to feel completely responsible for everything that happens at the scene, even things clearly out of their control. A few become so involved that their self-image is actually based on job performance.

Chronic stress at work plus an emotionally charged environment can lead to a state of exhaustion and irritability. Beware. That state can markedly decrease your effectiveness. Even some of the very best fire service personnel have had to leave EMS because of it.

Recognize Warning Signs

One of the best ways to manage chronic stress and prevent burnout is to be aware of the warning signs. The quicker they are spotted, the easier they are to remedy. The warning signs include (Figure 1-1):

◆ Irritability with coworkers, family, and friends.

◆ Inability to concentrate.

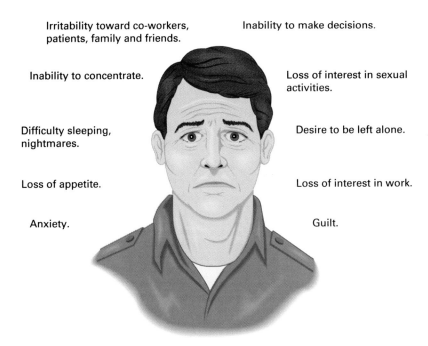

Irritability toward co-workers, patients, family and friends.

Inability to concentrate.

Difficulty sleeping, nightmares.

Loss of appetite.

Anxiety.

Inability to make decisions.

Loss of interest in sexual activities.

Desire to be left alone.

Loss of interest in work.

Guilt.

Figure 1-1 The warning signs of stress.

◆ Difficulty sleeping, nightmares, excessive sleeping.

◆ Anxiety.

◆ Inability to make decisions.

◆ Guilt.

◆ Loss of appetite.

◆ Loss of sexual desire.

◆ Isolation.

◆ Loss of interest in work.

In addition, the following general signs and symptoms have been identified with stress:

◆ *Cognitive*—confusion, inability to make judgments or decisions, loss of motivation, memory problems, loss of objectivity.

◆ *Psychological*—depression, excessive anger, negativism, hostility, defensiveness, mood swings, feelings of worthlessness.

◆ *Physical*—constant exhaustion, headaches, stomach problems, dizziness, pounding heart, high blood pressure, chest pain.

◆ *Behavioral*—overeating, increased use of drugs or alcohol, grinding teeth, hyperactivity, lack of energy.

◆ *Social*—frequent arguments, decreased ability to relate to patients.

Make Lifestyle Changes

Certain lifestyle changes can help you deal with chronic stress. Diet is one of them. Certain foods, such as sugar, fatty foods, caffeine, and alcohol increase the body's response to stress. So while at work, try to eat low-fat carbohydrates. Also, eat often but in small amounts.

Exercise more often (Figure 1-2). It offers all kinds of benefits, including physical release for pent-up emotions. It also breaks down the natural chemicals our bodies dump into our systems any-

Figure 1-2 As a First Responder, you must safeguard your own health.

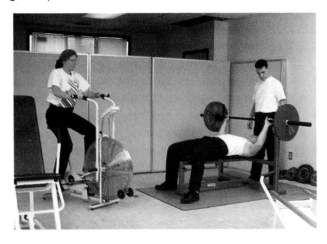

time we are under stress. Without exercise, these chemicals tend to build up, causing potentially harmful effects.

Finally, learn to relax. Meditation and visual imagery are helpful techniques. You also may want to try to cut loose a little bit. Watch a funny movie, read a good book, go dancing, or go to a concert.

Keep Balance in Your Life

Balance is an important principle of the world. We have all heard the terms "balance of nature," "balance of trade," and "balance of power." Yet, it is easy for First Responders to become unbalanced in their personal lives. One way to balance work, recreation, family, and health is by recognizing each role you play on a daily basis. For example, you not only have a role as a firefighter, you may also have a role as a parent, spouse, son or daughter, aunt or uncle, grandson or granddaughter, teacher or student, sibling, little league coach, or Girl Scout leader. It is critical for you to assess each and every one. Try this: Take a few minutes to list all your roles on paper. Most of us have at least five or six. After listing them, ask yourself this question: "Am I investing time and energy in one role at the expense of another?"

If you find you are out of balance, try the following:

◆ Each week write one or more goals to accomplish. Do it for each of your roles. This is a type of time management. Yet, most time-management tools do not consider all of our roles; they consider only our "work" role.

◆ Synergize roles, or combine actions, whenever possible. For example, if one of your goals is to exercise three times a week, try inviting your spouse or child. Swimming laps in a pool can be fun and aerobic when it becomes a family event. Or, when teaching a CPR class, have your spouse come in and be the "victim."

◆ It is important to recognize that your role as a fire service First Responder is not all there is to life! Has anyone ever heard of a firefighter whose last words were "I wish I had spent more time at the firehouse"? When you are on duty (at the station), give 100% of yourself. When you are off duty (away from the station), give 100% to the people you are with

and the activities you are involved in. In other words, wherever you are, be there.

◆ Finally, try to stay away from the firehouse. When you are off duty, stay off duty unless absolutely necessary.

It is important to remember that the support of your family and friends is essential to how well you manage stress. Keep in mind, though, that they suffer from stress related to your job, too. Their stress factors include the following:

◆ *Lack of understanding.* Families typically have little if any knowledge about prehospital emergency care.

◆ *Fear of separation or of being ignored.* Long hours can take their toll and increase your family's distress over your absences. You may hear, "the fire department is more important to you than your family!"

◆ *Worry about on-call situations.* Stress at home may increase because your family may focus on the danger you face when you respond to emergency calls.

◆ *Frustrated desire to share.* It may be too difficult for you to talk about what happened on certain calls. Even though your family and friends understand that, they may still feel frustrated in their desire to help and support you.

If at all possible, you can help to keep balance in your life by changing your work environment. Request work shifts that allow for more time to relax with family and friends. Ask for a rotation of duty to an assignment that is less stressful. Take periodic breaks to exercise and to support and encourage coworkers. If you are a volunteer, take some time off from responding to calls.

Seek Professional Help

Mental health professionals, social workers, and clergy can help you realize that your reactions— and your family's—are normal. They also can mobilize your best coping strategies and suggest more effective ways to deal with stress.

Critical Incident Stress Management (CISM)

A **critical incident** is any event that causes unusually strong emotions that interfere with your ability to function either during the incident or later. This type of stress requires aggressive and immediate management, including:

◆ Pre-incident stress education.

◆ On-scene peer support.

◆ One-on-one support.

◆ Disaster support services.

◆ Follow-up services.

◆ Spouse and family support.

◆ Community outreach programs.

◆ Other general health and welfare programs, such as wellness programs.

There are two basic critical incident stress management (CISM) techniques: debriefing and defusing.

Debriefing

The cornerstone of most CISM programs is called a **critical incident stress debriefing (CISD).** CISD combines a team of peer counselors with mental health professionals (Figure 1-3). It is successful because it helps rescuers vent their feelings quickly. Its nonthreatening environment also encourages rescuers to feel free to air their concerns and reactions.

CISD includes anyone involved in an incident— police, firefighters, EMS personnel, dispatchers, doctors, and so on. In some cases, it may also include their families.

Ideally, the debriefing is held within 24 to 72 hours of a critical incident. It is not an investi-

Figure 1-3 A critical incident stress debriefing (CISD).

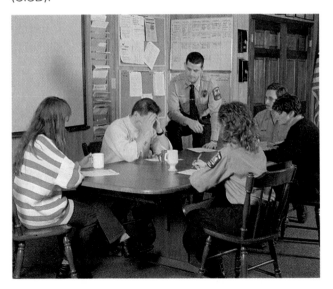

gation or an interrogation. Everything that is said at a debriefing is confidential. Rescuers are urged to explore any physical, mental, or emotional symptoms they are having. CISD counselors and mental health professionals then evaluate the information and offer suggestions on how to cope with the stress resulting from the incident.

After multiple-casualty incidents (such as earthquakes or explosions), a number of CISD meetings may be needed.

Defusing

Much shorter and less formal than a debriefing, a defusing is usually held within hours of the critical incident. It is attended only by those most directly involved and lasts only 30 to 45 minutes. A defusing gives rescuers a chance to vent their feelings and get information they may need before the larger group meets. It may either eliminate the need for a formal debriefing, or it may enhance a later debriefing.

Accessing CISD

Generally, your agency or organization will organize a CISD. Attend if you have been involved in:

◆ Serious injury or death of a rescuer in the line of duty.

◆ Multiple-casualty incident.

◆ Suicide of an emergency worker.

◆ An event that attracts media attention.

◆ Injury or death of someone you know.

◆ Any disaster.

◆ Injury or death of an infant or child.

Also access CISD after any event that has unusual impact on you. That may include an incident in which injury or death of a civilian was caused by a rescuer (an ambulance colliding with a car, for example). A death of a patient, child abuse or neglect, an event that threatens your life, or one that has distressing sights, sounds, or smells—all may be cause for accessing CISD.

Ask your instructor about the CISD programs available through your EMS system.

Death and Dying

Death and dying are inherent parts of emergency care. If you think about it, the fear of death is one of the most useless fears we have. Why? Death is one of the few things in life all of us will sooner

One of the most important actions any leader can take to minimize the stress related to emergency calls is to make work in the organization as stress free as possible. We know that our actual job of putting out fires, responding to hazardous materials spills, rescuing people from floods, and every other type of emergency causes stress on our employees. Why, then, would we want to pile even more stress on our workers through inefficient workplace practices—such as hazing rookies, not allowing firefighters to participate in decision-making on policy, and applying an autocratic leadership style around the firehouse? If, as a fire department manager, you are not directly involved in patient care, then you had better be directly involved in taking care of those people who are. Create a workplace environment that demonstrates care and respect for each individual. This is one of the most effective "anti-stress vaccines" available.

or later experience. If we are afraid of death, we might as well be afraid of gravity or breathing or "The Brady Bunch" reruns.

Be that as it may, it is most important to care for a dying patient's emotional needs. If the patient dies suddenly, his or her family becomes your patient. Be prepared to provide for their emotional needs and those of bystanders as well.

The Grieving Process

There are five general stages that dying patients—and those who are close to them—experience. The five stages are called the **grieving process.** Each person progresses through the stages at his or her own rate and in his or her own way.

Patients with nonfatal emergencies also may go through a grieving process. For example, a patient who loses both legs in a factory accident will grieve the loss of his limbs.

As a fire service First Responder, you will not witness all five stages during emergency care. For example, a critically injured patient who is aware that death is imminent may just begin the process. A terminally ill patient who is more prepared may be at the final "acceptance" stage. The key is to accept all emotions as real and necessary. Respond accordingly.

The stages of the grieving process occur as follows:

◆ *Denial ("Not me!")*. At first, the patient may refuse to accept the idea that death is near. This refusal creates a buffer between the shock of approaching death and the need to deal with the illness or injury. Families of dying patients often are at the denial stage.

◆ *Anger ("Why me?")*. Watch out. You may be the target of this anger. But remember that it is a normal part of the grieving process. Do not take it personally. Be tolerant. Try to understand, and use your best listening and communication skills.

◆ *Bargaining ("Okay, but first let me . . .")*. In the patient's mind a bargain, or agreement of sorts, will postpone death. For example, a patient may mentally determine that if he is allowed to live, he will patch up a long-standing break with his parents.

◆ *Depression ("Okay, but I haven't . . .")*. As reality settles in, the patient may become silent, distant, withdrawn, and sad. He usually is thinking about those he leaves behind and all the things left undone.

◆ *Acceptance ("Okay, I am not afraid.")*. Finally, the patient may appear to accept the fact that he is dying, though he is not happy about it. At this stage, the family usually needs more support than the patient does.

Dealing with the Dying Patient

It is one of your jobs to help a patient and his or her family through the grieving process. Keep in mind that they may progress through the stages of grief at different rates. Whatever stage they are in, their needs include dignity, respect, compassion, sharing, communication, privacy, and control. To help reduce their emotional burden, consider the following:

◆ *Do everything possible to maintain the patient's dignity.* Avoid negative statements about the patient's condition. Even an unresponsive patient may hear what you say and feel the fear in your words. Talk to the patient as if he or she is fully alert. Explain the care you are providing.

◆ *Show the greatest possible respect for the patient.* Do this especially when death is imminent. Families will be extra sensitive at this time. Even attitudes and unspoken messages are perceived. So explain what you are doing, and assure family members that you are making every possible effort to help the patient. It is important for them to know with certainty that you never simply "gave up."

♦ *Communicate.* Help the patient become oriented to the surroundings. If necessary, explain several times what happened and where. Explain who you are and what you and others are planning. Assure the patient that you are doing everything possible and that you will see that he or she gets to a hospital as quickly as possible. Without interrupting care, communicate the same message to the family. Explain any procedure you need to carry out. Answer their questions. Do not guess. Report only what you know to be true.

♦ *Allow family members to express rage, anger, and despair.* They should be able to scream, cry, or vent grief but in a way that is not dangerous to you or others. Be tolerant. If they vent their anger at you, do not get angry or hostile.

♦ *Listen with empathy.* Many dying people want messages delivered to survivors. Take notes. Assure the patient that you will do whatever you can to honor his or her requests. Then follow through on your promise. If necessary, stay with the family to listen to their concerns and answer their questions.

♦ *Do not give false assurances, but allow for some hope.* Be honest but tactful. If the patient asks if he is dying, do not confirm it. Patients who do the most poorly are often the ones who feel hopeless. Instead, say something like "We are doing everything we can. We need you to help us by not giving up." If the patient insists that death is imminent, say "That might be possible, but we can still try the best we can, can't we?"

♦ *Use a gentle tone of voice.* Be kind to both the patient and the family. Explain the scope of the injury and your medical care. When necessary, do so as gently and kindly as you can in terms they will understand.

♦ *Use a reassuring touch,* if appropriate.

♦ *Do what you can to comfort the family.* Arrange for them to briefly see or talk to the patient. However, do not interrupt your emergency care or delay transport.

♦ *If the patient is deceased* and no further medical interventions are indicated, and the family asks you to pray with them, do so. Call clergy or a chaplain, if the family requests it. Allow family members to touch or hold the body. The exception is at a crime scene. Never clean the patient or remove any blood from the patient or the crime scene itself. Finally, stay with the family until law enforcement, the medical examiner, coroner, or funeral home arrives.

SECTION

2 PREVENTING DISEASE TRANSMISSION

As a fire service First Responder, you will come in contact with patients who are sick. The following section will explain how diseases are transmitted and discuss the ones of most concern to the fire service First Responder. It also will describe ways for you to protect yourself.

How Diseases Are Transmitted

Diseases are caused by **pathogens,** microorganisms such as bacteria and viruses. An **infectious disease** is one that spreads from one person to another (Figure 1-4). It can spread *directly* through blood-to-blood contact (bloodborne), contact with open wounds or exposed tissues, and contact with the mucous membranes of the eyes and mouth. An infectious disease also can spread *indirectly* by way of a contaminated object, such as a needle, or by way of infected droplets inhaled into the respiratory tract (airborne).

Diseases also can be "vector-borne," or spread through contact with another organism. Examples include mosquito bites, which can spread malaria, or ticks, which can transmit Lyme disease.

Some pathogens are transmitted easily, such as the viruses that cause the common cold. Others need specific routes of contact. The tuberculosis bacteria, for example, is transmitted by droplets from a cough or sneeze of an infected patient. Poor nutrition, poor hygiene, crowded or unsanitary living conditions, and stress all make diseases easier to acquire.

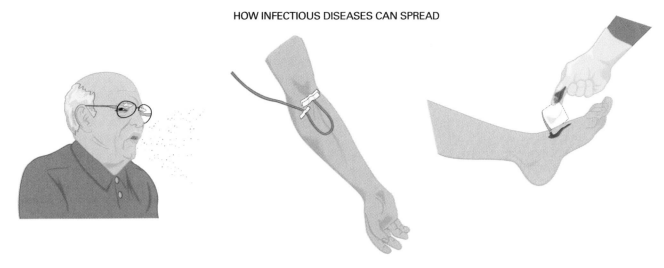

a. Droplet infection.　　b. Blood-to-blood contact.　　c. Open wounds/exposed tissue.

Figure 1-4　Infectious diseases can spread from one person to another.

In order to protect yourself, you must *always* make use of the appropriate body substance isolation (BSI) equipment, including barrier devices such as a pocket face mask, *every time* you ventilate a patient (Figure 1-5). Make sure barrier devices used for ventilation have a one-way valve that prevents fluid from backing up.

Diseases of Concern

As a fire service First Responder, every patient can potentially expose you to an infectious disease. Three diseases of most concern are described below.

Hepatitis B

Hepatitis B (HBV) is a potentially fatal virus directly affecting the liver. A serious disease that

Figure 1-5　A pocket face mask with one-way valve and carrying case.

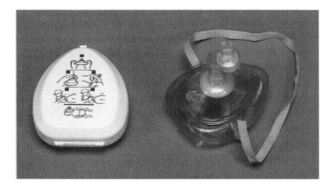

can last for months, HBV is contracted through blood and body fluids. A major source of the virus is the "chronic carrier," a person who carries the virus for years, often unaware that he or she is infected. When signs and symptoms do appear, they may include:

◆ Fatigue.

◆ Nausea.

◆ Loss of appetite.

◆ Abdominal pain.

◆ Headache.

◆ Fever.

◆ Yellowish color of the skin and whites of eyes.

The best defense against HBV infection is BSI equipment. The second best defense is the HBV vaccination, which most agencies and employers offer free of charge. If you suspect you have been exposed to HBV, report the incident to your infectious disease officer immediately or contact a physician or your local public health agency for care.

Tuberculosis

Tuberculosis (TB) is back with a vengeance. In fact, researchers are worried because of the development of new drug-resistant strains. The pathogen that causes TB is found in the lungs and other tissues of the infected patient. You can be infected from droplets in a patient's cough or from infected sputum. The signs and symptoms of TB include:

- Fever.
- Cough.
- Night sweats.
- Weight loss.

OSHA has adopted standards for rescuer protection against TB which include the use of special masks. One type of mask is called the **N-95 respirator** (Figure 1-6). Another type is called the **HEPA respirator,** or high efficiency particulate air respirator. Regardless of which mask your fire department chooses to use, it is critical that all First Responders wear one whenever a patient is suspected of having TB, or whenever a patient is coughing for an unknown reason.

Acquired Immune Deficiency Syndrome (AIDS)

Fortunately, acquired immune deficiency syndrome (AIDS) cannot be spread by touching the skin, coughing, sneezing, sharing eating utensils, or other indirect ways. *Transmission requires inti-*

Figure 1-6 Wear an N-95 respirator when you care for a patient with TB.

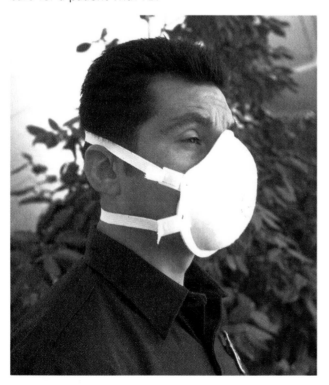

mate contact with the body fluids of infected persons. Infection may occur with:

- Sexual contact involving the exchange of semen, saliva, blood, urine, or feces.
- Infected needles.
- Infected blood or blood products, especially when it comes in contact with another person's eyes, mucous membranes, or broken skin.
- Mother to child during pregnancy, birth, or breast-feeding.

The human immunodeficiency virus (HIV) destroys the body's ability to fight infection. HIV can lead to AIDS. AIDS victims get infections caused by viruses, bacteria, parasites, and fungi—the same organisms that usually cause no harm in people with healthy immune systems. The infections involve many organs of the body, causing a countless array of signs and symptoms.

Not everyone infected by HIV develops AIDS. However, people who carry HIV are still able to spread the infection to others. Therefore, every patient you come in contact with could be infected with HIV or other diseases. To protect yourself, follow all the precautions described below at all times and with all patients.

Body Substance Isolation (BSI)

For many years, OSHA guidelines required all EMS personnel to take steps, or "universal precautions," to protect themselves against diseases transmitted through contact with blood. In the late 1980s, the Centers for Disease Control (CDC) published new guidelines. They make the assumption that *all blood and body fluids are infectious,* and therefore require all EMS personnel to practice a strict form of infection control with every patient. That strict form of infection control is called **body substance isolation (BSI).**

With BSI precautions, it is possible to take care of all patients safely, even those with infectious diseases. However, you must remember that it is not possible to tell if a patient is infectious by the way he looks, speaks, or acts. Treat all patients the same way. Always wear the proper BSI equipment with every patient.

BSI precautions include handwashing; proper cleaning, disinfection, or sterilization of equipment; and the use of BSI equipment.

Handwashing

Handwashing is the single most important thing you can do to prevent the spread of infection. According to the U.S. Public Health Service, most contaminants can be removed from the skin with 10 to 15 seconds of vigorous lathering and scrubbing with plain soap.

Always wash your hands after caring for a patient, even if you were wearing gloves. *For maximum protection, begin by removing all jewelry from your hands and arms.* Then lather up and rub together all surfaces of your hands. Pay attention to creases, crevices, and the areas between your fingers. Use a brush to scrub under and around your fingernails (Figure 1-7). (Note that it is a good idea for you to keep your nails short and unpolished.) If your hands are visibly soiled, spend more time washing them. Wash your wrists and forearms, too. Rinse thoroughly under a stream of water and dry well. Use a disposable towel if possible.

If you do not have access to soap and running water, you can use a foam or liquid washing agent. As soon as you can, wash your hands again using the procedure described above.

Cleaning Equipment

Cleaning, disinfecting, and sterilizing are related terms. **Cleaning** is simply the process of washing a soiled object with soap and water. **Disinfecting**

Figure 1-7 Washing your hands is the most important action you can take against the spread of infection.

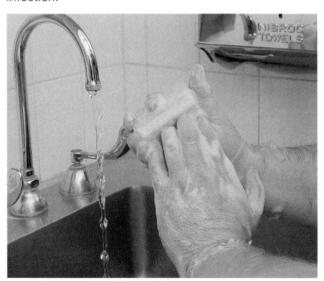

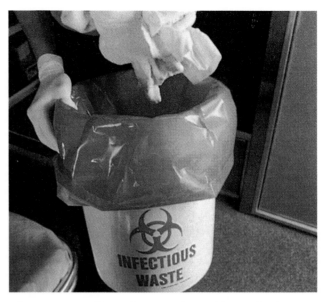

Figure 1-8 Discard contaminated items in the proper receptacle.

is cleaning plus using a chemical like alcohol or bleach to kill many of the microorganisms on an object. **Sterilizing** is a process in which a chemical or other substance (like superheated steam) kills all of the microorganisms on an object.

Generally, disinfection is used on items that make contact with intact skin, such as stethoscopes and blood pressure cuffs. Items that come in contact with open wounds or mucous membranes should be sterilized.

Whenever possible, use disposable equipment. Never reuse disposable items. Instead, place them in a plastic bag that is clearly labeled "infectious waste" (Figure 1-8). Then seal the bag. Disposable items used with patients who are known to have HBV or HIV should be double-bagged.

> **COMPANY OFFICER'S NOTE**
> Since you cannot be sure which patients may be infected with which diseases, use the following rule of thumb: All people have diseases. Therefore, double bag everything.

After each use, clean nondisposable equipment. Wash off all blood, mucus, tissue, and other residue. Be sure to wear a good pair of utility gloves while doing so. Then disinfect or sterilize it as per local protocols.

Wash items that do not normally touch the patient. Rinse them with clear water and dry thoroughly. Clean walls or window coverings in an ambulance or rescue vehicle when they get soiled. Then use a hospital-grade disinfectant or a solution of household bleach and water to clean up any blood or body fluids.

If your clothes get soiled with body fluids, remove, bag, and label them. Wash them in hot soapy water for at least 25 minutes. Do not mix contaminated and non-contaminated clothing in the washer. Take a hot shower yourself and rinse thoroughly.

BSI Equipment

Always use personal protective equipment (PPE) as a barrier against infection. Such items will keep you from coming into contact with a patient's blood and body fluids. They include eye protection, gloves, gowns, masks, and protection for the head and feet.

- *Eye protection.* Use eye shields to protect yourself from blood and body fluids splashing into your eyes. Several types are available. Clear plastic shields cover the eyes or the whole face. Safety glasses have side shields. If you wear prescription glasses, attach removable side shields. Form-fitting goggles are also available.

- *Gloves* (Figure 1-9). Wear high-quality vinyl or latex gloves whenever you care for a patient. Never reuse them. Put on a new pair for each patient to avoid exposing one patient to another's infection. Soiled gloves must be changed as soon as it is practical to do so. If a glove accidentally tears, remove it as soon as you can do so safely. Then wash your hands and replace the torn glove with a new one.

- *Gowns.* Wear a gown when there might be significant splashing of blood or body fluids. Generally, you will need a gown during childbirth or major injury. Whenever possible, use a disposable one. It also is recommended that you change your clothes if the gown gets soiled.

- *Masks.* Wear a disposable surgical-type face mask to protect against possible splatter of

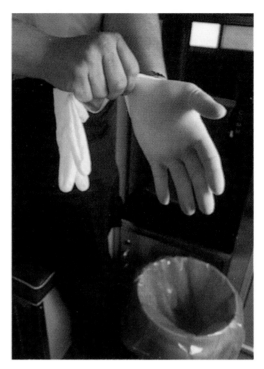

Figure 1-9 Wear protective gloves whenever you care for a patient.

blood or body fluids. An N-95 or HEPA respirator is recommended for use with suspected tuberculosis patients. An alternative is to place a properly fitted N-95 or HEPA respirator on your patient as well as on yourself.

- *Head and foot protection.* Under certain circumstances, head protection and shoe covers may be required to protect you from excessive splashing or contamination from fluids. Hospital head and footwear usually worn in the hospital operating room may be one type of protective gear used for this purpose. Structural firefighting gear, such as impervious boots and helmets with face shields, also may be appropriate. Always check local protocols.

Use BSI equipment yourself and be sure to remind other EMS personnel at the scene to wear it, too. Make gloves and other PPE available to others who arrive to help.

Immunizations

Before you begin providing First Responder care, have a physician make sure you are adequately protected against common infectious diseases.

Health-care workers wearing latex gloves on a daily basis have a risk of developing latex allergy that is greater than the general population. Unfortunately, it is not possible to predict when and if any individual will develop a latex allergy. The most common symptom is a poison ivy-like rash on the hands. However, serious allergic reactions—including death—have occurred in a number of cases.

Fire service First Responders can avoid this problem by using non-latex gloves, such as those made of nitrile. However, if latex gloves are used as the appropriate protection, they should be reduced-protein, powder-free latex gloves. Note that powder used as a lubricant in some gloves can increase exposure to the allergy.

If you use latex gloves, always ask your patients if they are allergic to latex prior to touching them, if possible. Several groups are at high risk for latex allergy, including children with serious congenital defects, such as spina bifida, and individuals who have already been sensitized.

The following immunizations are recommended for active-duty fire service First Responders:

◆ Tetanus prophylaxis (every 10 years).

◆ Hepatitis B vaccine.

◆ Influenza vaccine (every year).

◆ Polio.

◆ Rubella (German measles).

◆ Measles.

◆ Mumps.

Because some immunizations offer only partial protection, have your physician verify your immune status against rubella, measles, and mumps. Remember always practice BSI precautions, even after being vaccinated.

Have a tuberculin skin (tine) test at least once every year you are on duty. It will tell you if you have been exposed to TB. If you have been exposed, you will require more frequent testing. Your agency's medical director or your physician can advise you.

Reporting Exposures

Immediately report any suspected exposure to blood or body fluids to your infectious disease officer, to medical control, and to your immediate supervisor, especially if the patient is HIV-positive, has hepatitis B, or is in a high-risk category for infection. Include in your report the date and time of the exposure, the type of body fluid involved, the amount, and details of the incident. State laws vary, so be sure to follow all local protocols.

SECTION 3
SCENE SAFETY

The number-one priority at each and every scene is to protect yourself. Be part of the solution, not part of the problem.

The only valid assumption regarding scene safety is to assume the worst. We all know there is absolutely no place on the fireground for the "hero mentality." The same is true on any EMS scene. No scene should ever be considered "secure" as long as there are people involved. That means every scene! Remember, it's people who shoot guns, wield knives, drive vehicles, and swing bats. As an instructor once said, "I never thought much of the courage of a lion-tamer. Inside the cage he is at least safe from people."

As you approach a scene, turn off your lights and siren to avoid broadcasting your arrival, if it is safe to do so. Take a good look at the neighborhood. If possible, do not park directly in front of the call address. This is so you can size up the scene unnoticed and save a place for an ambulance to park.

Then decide whether or not it is safe to approach the patient. If any of the following exists on scene, you may need to call for help:

◆ Motor-vehicle or airplane crashes.

◆ Presence of toxic substances or low levels of oxygen.

- Crime scenes.
- Presence of a weapon of any kind.
- Possible drug or alcohol use.
- Arguing, threats, violent behavior, broken glass, overturned furniture.
- Unstable surfaces, such as water and ice.
- Any type of entrapment.

While each emergency scene is unique, a general rule applies to all. *If the scene is unsafe, make it safe before you enter.* Otherwise, wait for help to arrive. Specialized personnel will have the training, equipment, and protective gear needed to enter an unstable scene safely.

Once a scene is secure, take measures to protect the patient from hazards. That includes fire, structural instability, gasoline leaks, chemical spills, oncoming traffic, and extremes in temperature. Bystanders should also be protected from illness or injury.

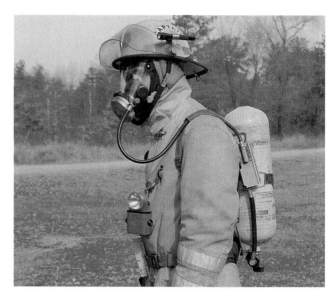

Figure 1-10 A self-contained breathing apparatus (SCBA).

In general, specialized team members should wear protective clothing, such as a self-contained breathing apparatus (Figure 1-10) and a "hazmat" suit (Figure 1-11). Although it is important for you to learn how to access your local hazmat team, you should at least be trained to the hazmat "awareness" level.

COMPANY OFFICER'S NOTE

At every EMS scene, it is important for you to remember to perform a size up that is similar to the one performed when arriving at a burning building. Just like a size up for a reported structure fire, this size up can begin at the time of dispatch. Is it day or night? Is it during the week or on the weekend or a holiday, when alcohol or drugs may be involved or a large gathering of people? Does the dispatcher report the call as an "unknown problem?" Could this be a potential crime scene? Is there the possibility of violence? If so, is law enforcement en route? If this is a reported car crash, is it on a 65-mph (100 km/h) interstate, which requires additional resources "just in case," or is it on a town street with a posted speed limit of 25 mph (40 km/h)? Remember, the scene size-up is important in accomplishing your number one objective: your safety!

Figure 1-11 Typical hazardous materials protective suit.

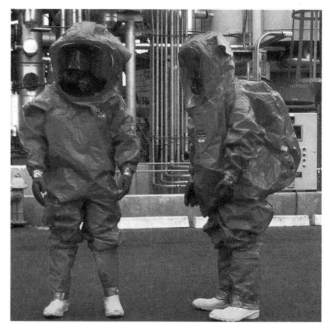

Hazardous Materials

Do not enter a hazardous materials scene. Call a specialized team of rescuers to secure the scene first. Provide emergency care only after the scene is safe and the patient has been decontaminated.

Motor-Vehicle Collisions

Some car crashes lead to situations that threaten the life of both patients and rescuers. For example:

◆ Downed power lines or other potential sources of electrocution.

◆ Fire or the potential for fire such as leaking gasoline.

◆ Explosion or the potential for explosion.

◆ Hazardous materials.

◆ Oncoming traffic.

◆ Unstable vehicles.

When there is life-threatening danger on scene, call for specially trained personnel *before you enter*. Also call for special teams when a complex or extensive rescue is needed. Once a scene is safe, make sure you are wearing the proper personal protective equipment before you enter, including turnout gear, puncture-resistant gloves with latex or non-latex gloves underneath, helmet, and eye protection (Figure 1-12). Follow local protocols.

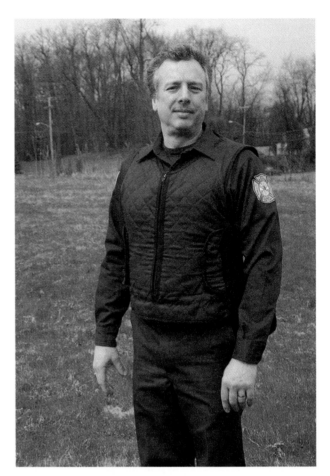

Figure 1-13 Body armor, or bullet-proof vest.

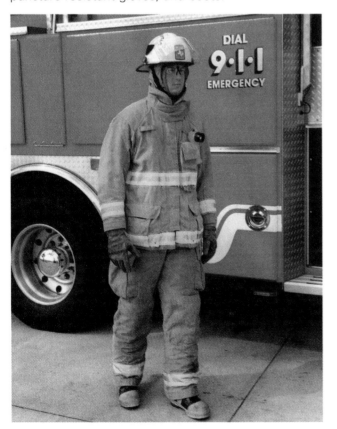

Figure 1-12 Turnout gear, plus helmet, eyewear, puncture-resistant gloves, and boots.

Initial positioning of rescue vehicles can help in protecting fire department personnel from oncoming traffic. Check local protocols or standard operating procedures for information on proper apparatus positioning.

Violence

You may face violence without warning, from a patient, bystander, or perpetrator of a crime. If you suspect potential violence, call law enforcement before you enter the scene. Never enter the scene to give patient care until it has been adequately controlled by the police.

Always call for law enforcement in cases of domestic disputes, street or gang fights, bar fights, potential suicides, crime scenes, and incidents involving angry family or bystanders. Remember, violence does not only occur in dark alleys. Case in point: violence is the leading cause of trauma in the workplace.

No matter where you work, consider using **body armor** (Figure 1-13). It is made of Kevlar™

or other synthetic materials that resist penetration by bullets. The amount of protection it offers depends on the tightness of the weave and the number of layers. While it will protect you, body armor will not make you invincible. You are still vulnerable in the areas not covered, and you can still be killed by the blunt force of a bullet, even if it does not penetrate the armor. Never take chances you would normally avoid just because you are wearing armor.

If you need to treat patients at a crime scene, you must preserve the chain of evidence needed for investigation and prosecution. A general rule is to avoid disturbing the scene unless absolutely necessary for medical care. Basic guidelines include:

◆ Never wipe away blood. It can be used as evidence.

◆ Touch only what you need to touch to provide patient care.

◆ Move only what you need to move to protect the patient and to provide proper care.

◆ Do not use the telephone unless the police give you permission to do so.

◆ Observe and document anything unusual at the scene.

◆ If possible, do not cut through holes in the patient's clothing. The holes could have been caused by bullets or other penetrating weapons.

◆ Do not cut through any knot in a rope or tie. Knots are used as evidence. Cut the rope or tie somewhere away from the knot.

◆ If the crime is rape, attempt to discourage the patient from washing, changing clothes, using the bathroom, or taking anything by mouth. Any of these actions could damage valuable evidence.

◆ ON SCENE FOLLOW-UP

At the beginning of this chapter, you read that fire service First Responders were at a potentially dangerous scene. To see how chapter skills apply to this emergency, read the following. It describes how the call was completed.

SCENE SIZE-UP (CONTINUED)

My partner and I looked at each other. We decided to move our vehicle away from the front of the building and radio dispatch to double check that the police had given us the "OK" to enter the building.

We moved our vehicle out of sight, and waited. Finally, dispatch informed us that the police had secured the scene. Meanwhile, my partner tapped me on the shoulder and pointed to the house. I saw an officer standing outside the front door waving at us. We approached the scene, but with caution.

The officer told us that two brothers had been in a fist fight and that both had consumed "too much nitwit." My partner smiled and told me that "nitwit" was street jargon for alcohol. One of the brothers said his hand went through a window. Both of the brothers appeared to be intoxicated.

INITIAL ASSESSMENT

After we put on eye protection and latex-free gloves, we introduced ourselves to Hubert, the brother who needed medical help. He seemed calm. Hubert had moderate bleeding from his left forearm. His airway and breathing were good. He denied any other injuries or falls.

PHYSICAL EXAMINATION

We decided to do a physical exam anyway. Sometimes people get into fights and get so excited that they don't know they're hurt (especially when they've had too much "nitwit"). Since there were two of us, my partner controlled the bleeding while I checked Hubert's head, neck, chest, abdomen, and extremities.

While we were waiting for an ambulance, Hubert's brother became loud and abusive to the police. We had the patient walk outside with us to get away from the potential danger. There we checked his pulse and respirations.

PATIENT HISTORY

Hubert admitted to drinking six or eight cans of beer before the fight started. He told us that he had asthma, but wasn't feeling any respiratory distress or problems. He took an inhaler for his asthma, but didn't have it with him. He continued to deny any injuries other than the cut to his forearm.

ONGOING ASSESSMENT

We reassessed Hubert's airway and breathing. They were okay. Hubert didn't have any changes in mental status. The bleeding was controlled and the bandages were secure. We didn't get to recheck the vitals before the ambulance arrived.

PATIENT HAND-OFF

We advised the EMTs:

"The patient's name is Hubert. He's a 22-year-old male who has sustained a laceration to his left forearm from going through a window. The wound has been dressed and bandaged. The bleeding was moderate and was easily controlled. Hubert has been drinking but has been alert and oriented throughout the call. His airway and breathing are good. He denies any other injuries. He has a history of asthma and uses an inhaler, which he doesn't have with him. The physical exam was negative for injuries anywhere other than his arm. His pulse is 82, strong, and regular. His respirations are 20 and adequate. We were about to recheck his vitals as you pulled up."

Life safety—first yours and then your patient's—are your top priorities. Without them, you cannot be an effective First Responder. Throughout this textbook, you will find reminders about taking BSI and other safety precautions. Make note of them.

Chapter Review

Unfortunately for all rescue workers, television and movies have led the public to believe that it is okay for fire and EMS personnel to rush into calls without regard for their safety, fostering a "hero mentality." Nothing could be further from the truth. As a fire service First Responder, you are there to keep the problem from getting worse. If you become injured or ill, you become part of that problem, which helps no one.

One of the most important factors to be considered in the first 10 minutes of a call is your own personal safety. Practice body substance isolation (BSI) precautions on every call. And always remain alert for violence, hazardous materials, and other unsafe conditions.

You owe it to yourself to stay safe when responding to every call, regardless if it is a structure fire or an EMS call. You also owe it to your family, your department, and to the community you serve. Although unforeseen events do occur on every emergency scene, it is your personal responsibility—not your company officer's, not your fire chief's, and not your partner's—to take the necessary precautions to protect yourself. It is a foolhardy person who declares it "my duty" to help a citizen without first protecting himself and the other rescuers with him.

Do not underestimate the importance of the information in this chapter. There will be reminders in every chapter in this book.

FIRE COMPANY REVIEW

Page references where answers may be found or supported are provided at the end of each question.

Section 1

1. What are three techniques you can use to help you avoid responses like nausea or fainting in an emergency situation? (p. 3)

2. What are the five stages of the grieving process? (p. 7)

3. What can you do to help a dying patient, in addition to providing medical care? (pp. 7–8)

4. What are five signs of chronic stress and burnout? (pp. 3–4)

5. What are some of the negative feelings a First Responder's family may have about the job? (p. 5)

6. What are three examples of situations that may cause critical incident stress? (p. 6)

7. What is a critical incident stress debriefing (CISD)? (p. 6)

Section 2

8. How does an infectious disease spread from person to person? (pp. 8–9)

9. What equipment is needed to take BSI precautions? (p. 12)

Section 3

10. What general rule applies to all unsafe emergency scenes? (p. 13)

EMS Safety: Techniques and Applications. Federal Emergency Management Agency/U.S. Fire Administration, FA-144. Washington, D.C.: April 1994.

Kübler-Ross, E. *On Death and Dying.* New York: Collier Books/Macmillan, 1969.

West, K.H. *Infectious Disease Handbook for Emergency Care Personnel.* Philadelphia: J.B. Lippincott, 1987.

Wieder, M.A., ed. *Fire Department Pumping Apparatus Driver/Operator,* Eighth Edition. Stillwater, OK: International Fire Service Training Association, 1999.

Wieder, M.A., ed. *Hazardous Materials for First Responders,* Second Edition. Stillwater, OK: International Fire Service Training Association, 1994.

Wieder, M.A., ed. *Principles of Extrication.* Stillwater, OK: International Fire Service Training Association, 1990.

Zimmerman, L., M. Neuman, and D. Jurewicz. *Infection Control for Prehospital Providers,* Second Edition. Grand Rapids, MI: Mercy Ambulance, 1993.

THE CISM PROCESS

CRITICAL INCIDENT OCCURS
Produces strong emotional response in emergency workers

↓

NEED FOR CISM RECOGNIZED
Usually the company officer arranges for CISM, but any emergency worker involved in incident can request one

↓

CISD SCHEDULED
Usually held within 24 to 72 hours of incident

↓

THE CISD
Participants include those involved in incident, trained peer counselors, mental health professionals; process involves the following seven phases:

↓

PHASE 1: INTRODUCTION
Sets goals for the CISD. Assures confidentiality.

↓

PHASE 2: FACTS
Sets out details of what occurred at the incident

↓

PHASE 3: FEELINGS
Encourages participants to explore feelings the incident raised in them

↓

PHASE 4: SYMPTOMS
Encourages participants to note any physical reactions the incident may have caused in them

↓

PHASE 5: TEACHING
Allows professionals to help participants sort through feelings; provides opportunity to reinforce that extreme reactions are normal in such situations

↓

PHASE 6: RE-ENTRY
Offers suggestions for coping after the CISD; may include an action plan with goals and activities to reduce stress

↓

PHASE 7: FOLLOW-UP
Explores how participants are coping months or weeks later

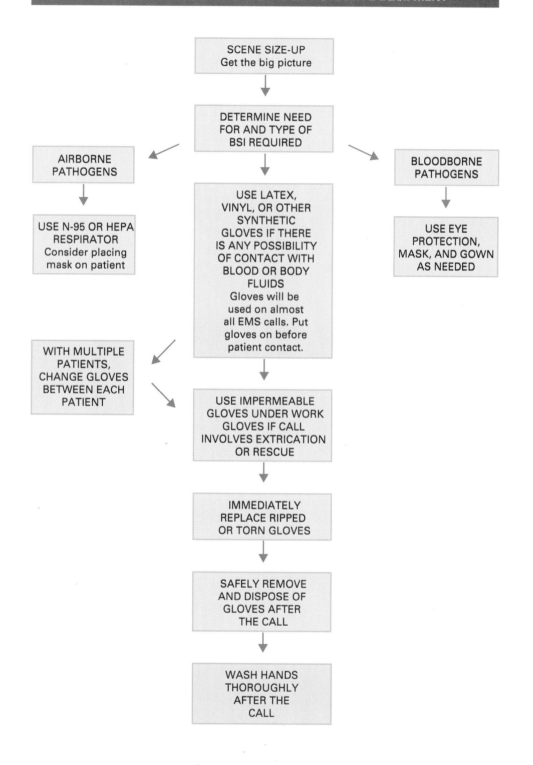

Circulation

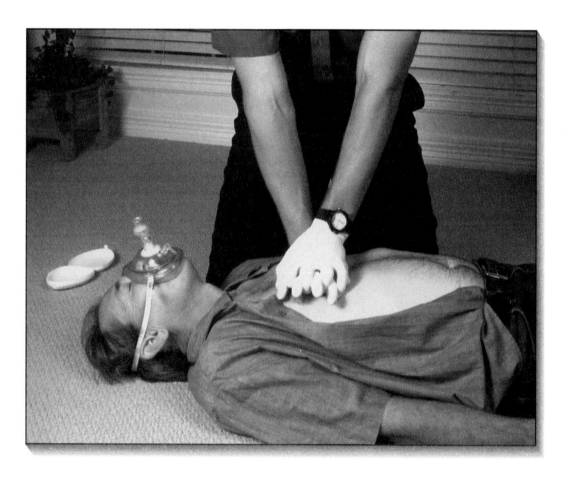

I **NTRODUCTION** *Heart disease takes the lives of about 600,000 Americans each year. Included in that total are the 350,000 people a year—about 1,000 a day—that suffer from sudden cardiac arrest. Only one in 20 survive. The people who can be saved need immediate CPR followed by advanced medical care, including defibrillation, within 8 to 10 minutes of collapse.*

But even with CPR, many patients will not live. They may have been without a pulse or breathing for too long or cardiac arrest may have caused irreversible damage to the heart. Please do not let that discourage you. Emergency care in the field is still critical to saving many lives. And today's new hospital techniques often help to reverse the crippling effects of heart attack or cardiac arrest.

Note that several studies have shown that you can lose your CPR skills unless you have frequent practice and retraining. Retraining should occur every one to two years.

OBJECTIVES

Cognitive, affective, and psychomotor objectives are from the U.S. DOT's "First Responder: National Standard Curriculum." Enrichment objectives, if any, identify supplemental material.

Cognitive

4-1.1 List the reasons for the heart to stop beating. (p. 26)

4-1.2 Define the components of cardiopulmonary resuscitation. (p. 27)

4-1.3 Describe each link in the chain of survival and how it relates to the EMS system. (pp. 26–27)

4-1.4 List the steps of one-rescuer adult CPR. (pp. 31–35)

4-1.5 Describe the technique of external chest compressions on an adult patient. (pp. 29–31)

4-1.6 Describe the technique of external chest compressions on an infant. (pp. 38–42)

4-1.7 Describe the technique of external chest compressions on a child. (pp. 38–42)

4-1.8 Explain when the First Responder is able to stop CPR. (pp. 36–37)

4-1.9 List the steps of two-rescuer adult CPR. (pp. 35–37)

4-1.10 List the steps of infant CPR. (pp. 40–42)

4-1.11 List the steps of child CPR. (pp. 40–42)

Affective

4-1.12 Respond to the feelings that the family of a patient may be having during a cardiac event. (p. 27)

4-1.13 Demonstrate a caring attitude towards patients with cardiac events who request emergency medical services. (p. 27)

4-1.14 Place the interests of the patient with a cardiac event as the foremost consideration when making any and all patient care decisions. (p. 27)

4-1.15 Communicate with empathy with family members and friends of the patient with a cardiac event. (p. 27)

Psychomotor

4-1.16 Demonstrate the proper technique of chest compressions on an adult. (pp. 29–31)

4-1.17 Demonstrate the proper technique of chest compressions on a child. (pp. 40–42)

4-1.18 Demonstrate the proper technique of chest compressions on an infant. (pp. 40–42)

4-1.19 Demonstrate the steps of adult one rescuer CPR. (pp. 31–35)

4-1.20 Demonstrate the steps of adult two rescuer CPR. (pp. 35–37)

4-1.21 Demonstrate child CPR. (pp. 40–42)

4-1.22 Demonstrate infant CPR. (pp. 40–42)

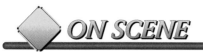

ON SCENE

Our F.A.S.T. (First Aid Stabilization Team) unit was dispatched on an EMS assist because the closest ambulance was unavailable. The call was for a possible heart attack. As I climbed into our vehicle, I realized that time would really count.

SCENE SIZE-UP

There were three of us assigned to the F.A.S.T unit. Being the senior officer, I sized up the scene carefully from the cab before we got out. I reminded the others to put on their BSI equipment. An elderly man met us half-way to the door and stated, "You better hurry up. They're doing CPR on my brother."

INITIAL ASSESSMENT

Inside the home, we observed a woman performing CPR on an older gentleman. The woman seemed to be doing pretty well but she was getting tired. My crew approached and took over. Checking the patient's ABCs (airway, breathing, and circulation), we found no pulse or respirations. We continued with CPR.

> *CPR is an important skill for the First Responder. Though needed in only a small percentage of calls, when it is used, it is vitally important. In the scenario described above, the firefighters have begun CPR. How long do you think they should continue? Could CPR injure the patient? Will the patient live? Consider these questions as you read this chapter.*

1   THE CIRCULATORY SYSTEM

The circulatory system is responsible for delivering oxygen and nutrients to the body's tissues. It also is responsible for removing waste from the tissues. Its basic components are the heart, arteries, veins, capillaries, and blood.

The heart is a hollow, muscular organ about the size of a fist. It lies in the lower left central region of the chest between the lungs. It is protected in the front by the ribs and sternum (breastbone). In the back it is protected by the spinal column. The heart contains four chambers. The two upper ones are the left and right atria. The two lower ones are the left and right ventricles. The septum (a wall) divides the right side of the heart from the left side. The heart also contains several one-way valves that keep blood flowing in the correct direction.

The circulatory system contains blood vessels. These vessels transport blood throughout the body. Arteries transport blood away from the heart. Veins carry blood back to the heart. The tiny capillaries allow for the exchange of gases and nutrients between the blood and the cells of the body.

How the Heart Works

The heart is like a two-sided pump (Figure 2-1). The left side receives oxygenated blood from the lungs and pumps it to all parts of the body. The right side receives blood from the body and then pumps it to the lungs to be reoxygenated.

The blood is kept under pressure and in constant circulation by the heart's pumping action. In a healthy adult at rest, the heart contracts between 60 and 80 times per minute. The pulse is a sign of the pressure exerted during each contraction of the heart. Every time the heart pumps, a wave of blood is sent through the arteries. That wave is

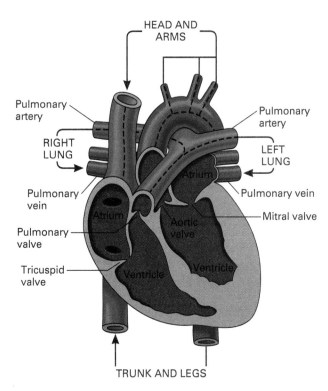

HEAD AND ARMS

Pulmonary artery

RIGHT LUNG

Pulmonary artery

LEFT LUNG

Pulmonary vein

Atrium

Atrium

Pulmonary vein

Mitral valve

Aortic valve

Pulmonary valve

Tricuspid valve

Ventricle

Ventricle

TRUNK AND LEGS

RIGHT HEART:
Receives blood from
the body and pumps
it through the pulmonary
artery to the lungs where
it picks up fresh oxygen.

LEFT HEART:
Receives oxygen-full
blood from the lungs
and pumps it through
the aorta to the body.

Figure 2-1 Cross-section of the heart.

felt as a pulse. It can be palpated, or felt, most easily where a large artery lies over a bone close to the skin. Sites include: the carotid pulse in the neck, the brachial pulse in underside of the upper arm, the radial pulse in the thumb side of the wrist, and the femoral pulse in the upper thigh.

The pulse is felt most easily over the carotid artery on either side of the neck. The carotid artery should be palpated (felt) first when a patient is unresponsive. The radial artery on the thumb side of the inner surface of the wrist is also easy to feel. It should be palpated first when the patient is responsive.

The heart, lungs, and brain work together closely to sustain life. The smooth functioning of each is critical to the others. When one organ cannot perform properly, the other two are handicapped. If one fails, the other two soon will follow.

When the Heart Stops

Clinical death occurs when a patient is in **respiratory arrest** and **cardiac arrest.** Immediate

CPR slows the death process and is critical for patient survival. However, if a patient is clinically dead for 4 to 6 minutes, brain cells begin to die. After 8 to 10 minutes without a pulse, irreversible damage occurs to the brain, regardless of how well CPR is performed.

There are many reasons why a heart will stop. They include heart disease, stroke, allergic reaction, diabetes, prolonged seizures, and other medical conditions. The heart also may stop because of a serious injury. In infants and children, respiratory problems are the most common cause of cardiac arrest. This is why airway care is so important in young patients.

COMPANY OFFICER'S NOTE

Remember: A heart attack and cardiac arrest are not the same! A person having a heart attack will most likely be conscious and talking to you when you arrive on scene. However, it is important for you to know that 30% of heart-attack victims will be in cardiac arrest when the fire department First Responder arrives on scene. Therefore, hope for the best (a conscious, alive, and talking patient), but be prepared for the worst (an unconscious, non-breathing, and pulseless patient in cardiac arrest).

The patient in respiratory and cardiac arrest has the best chance of surviving if all of the links in the **chain of survival** come together. This "chain" as identified by the American Heart Association (AHA) contains four links:

◆ *Early access.* Lay people must activate the EMS system immediately. The use of a universal access number (9-1-1, for example) helps to speed system access.

◆ *Early CPR.* Family members, citizens, and First Responders must be trained in CPR and begin as soon as possible. CPR will help to sustain life until the next step.

◆ *Early defibrillation.* Defibrillation is the process by which an electrical current is sent to the heart to correct fatal heart rhythms. The earlier defibrillation can be performed, the better.

◆ *Early advanced care.* Advanced care, or the administration of medications and other advanced therapies, must start as soon as possible. This can be done by paramedics at the scene or by prompt transportation to the emergency department.

As a First Responder, you have an important role. You can provide early CPR and, if permitted in your area, defibrillation.

The principle of CPR is to oxygenate and circulate the blood of the patient until defibrillation and advanced care can be given. Any delay in starting CPR increases the chances of nervous system damage and death. The faster the response, the better the patient's chances are. Survival rates improve when the time between arrest and the delivery of defibrillation and other advanced measures is short.

FIRE DRILL

When responding to a structure fire, it is important to get equipment and manpower on scene as quickly as possible. In fact, the time of ignition of a fire to flashover is about eight minutes (time-temperature curve). Therefore, it is critical to assess, perform rescue, and ventilate as soon as possible in order to avoid "irreversible" damage to the structure. Similarly, it is just as critical to assess, perform rescue breathing and chest compressions, and defibrillate within eight minutes to avoid irreversible damage to the structure of the brain.

---

2 CARDIOPULMONARY RESUSCITATION (CPR)

According to the American Heart Association (AHA), proper assessment of the patient's airway, breathing, and circulation is critical to successful CPR. The AHA also states that no patient should undergo the intrusive procedures of CPR until need is clearly established.

You can establish the need for CPR by determining that the patient is unresponsive, breathless, and pulseless.

To perform CPR, you must maintain an open airway, provide artificial ventilation, and provide artificial circulation by means of chest compressions.

CPR must begin as soon as possible and continue until the:

◆ First Responder is exhausted and is unable to continue.

◆ Patient is turned over to another trained rescuer or the hospital staff.

◆ Patient is resuscitated.

◆ Patient has been declared dead by a proper authority.

A cardiac event is very serious. Without your interventions, the patient may not survive. So remember to place his or her interests first. And be sure to demonstrate a caring attitude. When possible, respond to the feelings of the patient's family and friends with empathy.

Steps Preceding CPR

Before providing CPR to a patient, you must first (Figure 2-2):

◆ Determine unresponsiveness.

◆ Determine breathlessness.

◆ Determine pulselessness.

To determine unresponsiveness, tap or gently shake the patient and shout, "Are you okay?" If the patient does not respond, and if you are alone, immediately activate the EMS system for an adult (after one minute of care for an infant or child). This increases the patient's chances of early defibrillation and early advanced care. Then continue with your assessment.

If, after opening the patient's airway, you determine breathlessness, provide artificial ventilation. Provide supplemental oxygen, if you are allowed, by attaching it to your pocket face mask. The oxygen should flow at 15–25 liters per minute.

To determine pulselessness, find the carotid artery pulse point (Figure 2-3):

1. **Place two fingers on the larynx ("Adam's apple").**

Steps Preceding CPR

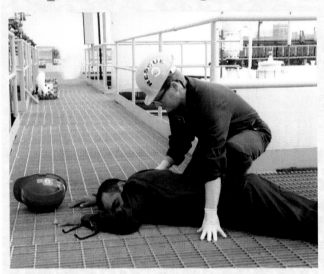

Figure 2-2a Determine unresponsiveness.

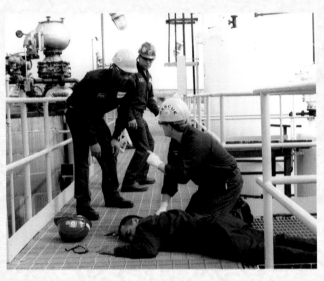

Figure 2-2b Be sure EMS has been activated.

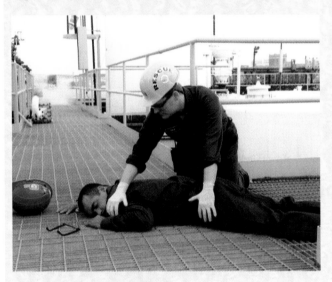

Figure 2-2c Position the patient. He or she should be supine on a firm, flat surface.

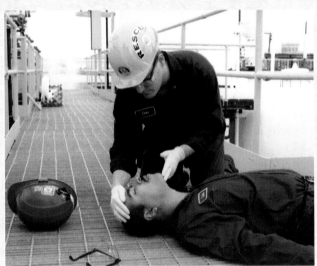

Figure 2-2d Open the airway.

2. **Slide your fingers to the side.** Stop in the groove between the larynx and the large neck muscle.

3. **Feel for the pulse.** Press for 5 to 10 seconds, gently enough to avoid compressing the artery. Do not use your thumb. Do not rest your hand across the patient's throat.

If the patient has a pulse—even a weak or irregular one, do not begin chest compressions.

You could cause serious problems. Monitor the pulse frequently. If you find the patient has no pulse, assume that he or she is in cardiac arrest. Begin CPR immediately.

Note that to perform CPR correctly, your patient must be in a supine position on a firm, flat surface such as the floor or a backboard.

You may wish to refer to the CPR summary, Figure 2-4, as you read the rest of this chapter.

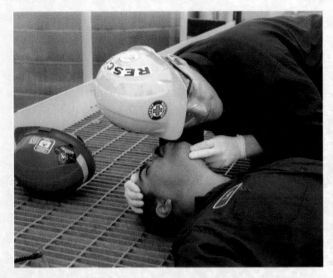

Figure 2-2e Determine breathlessness.

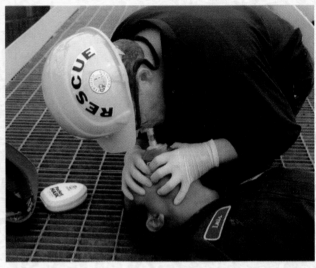

Figure 2-2f Provide artificial ventilation.

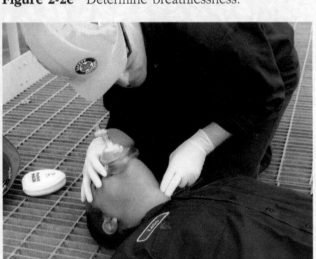

Figure 2-2g Determine pulselessness.

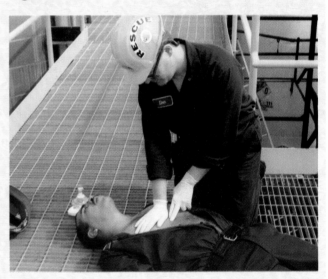

Figure 2-2h Bare the chest, locate the proper hand position, and begin CPR.

CPR for Adults

CPR involves a combination of skills. When a patient's heart has stopped, artificial ventilation alone cannot help the patient. Chest compressions also must be used to circulate the oxygen in the blood.

Chest compressions consist of rhythmic, repeated pressure over the lower half of the sternum. They cause blood to circulate as a result of the build-up of pressure in the chest cavity. When combined with artificial ventilation, they provide enough blood circulation to maintain life for a short time.

To perform chest compressions, take BSI precautions. Then follow these steps:

1. **Position the patient.** He or she must be supine on a firm, flat surface such as the floor.

2. **Uncover the chest.** Remove the patient's shirt or blouse. Do not waste time unbuttoning it.

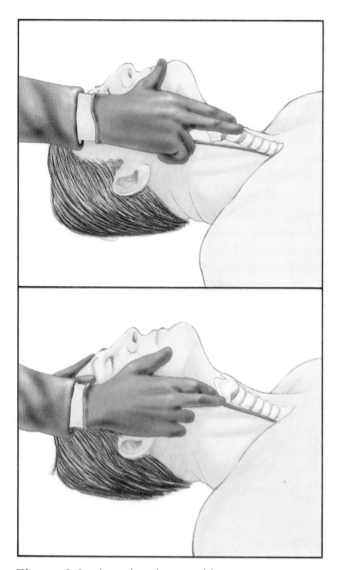

Figure 2-3 Locating the carotid artery.

Rip it open or pull it up. Cut a woman's bra in two or slip it up to her neck.

3. **Get in position.** Kneel close to the patient's side. Have your knees about as wide as your shoulders.

4. **Locate the xiphoid process** (Figure 2-5). First feel the lower margin of the rib cage on the side nearest you. Use the middle and index fingers of your hand, the one closest to the patient's feet. Then run your fingers along the rib cage to the notch where the ribs meet the sternum in the center of the lower chest.

5. **Locate the compression site** (Figure 2-6). Place your middle finger on the xiphoid process (the notch). Put your index finger of the same hand on the lower end of the patient's sternum. Then place the heel of your other hand alongside your fingers. There should be two finger widths between the tip of the sternum and the place where you rest the heel of your hand. When you apply pressure at this point, the sternum is flexible enough to be compressed without breaking. (A fracture of the sternum or the ribs can cut the heart, lungs, or liver.)

6. **Position your hands.** Put your free hand on top of the hand that is on the sternum. Your hands should be parallel. Extend or interlace your fingers to hold them off the chest wall. If your fingers rest against the chest wall during compressions, you increase the chance of separating and injuring the patient's ribs. (An alternative position for large hands and hands or wrists with arthritis is to use your free hand to grasp the wrist of the hand on the patient's sternum.)

7. **Position your shoulders.** Put them directly over your hands.

8. **Perform chest compressions.** Keeping your arms straight and your elbows locked. Your shoulders should be directly over the patient's chest. Compress the chest while bending or pivoting from the hips. Apply firm, heavy pressure. Depress the sternum 1.5 to 2 inches (40 mm to 55 mm) on an adult. Be sure the thrust is straight down into the sternum. If it is not, compressions may not be centered properly on the chest and part of the force of the thrust will be lost.

   Using the weight of your body, deliver smooth compressions without jerking or jabbing. If necessary, add force to the thrusts with your shoulders. Never add force with your arms—the force is too great and could fracture the sternum. Compressions should be 50% of the cycle. That is, the compression and release time should be about equal.

9. **Completely release pressure after each compression.** Let the sternum return to its normal position, and allow blood to flow back into the chest and heart. If you do not release all pressure, blood will not circulate properly. Do not lift or move your hands in any way.

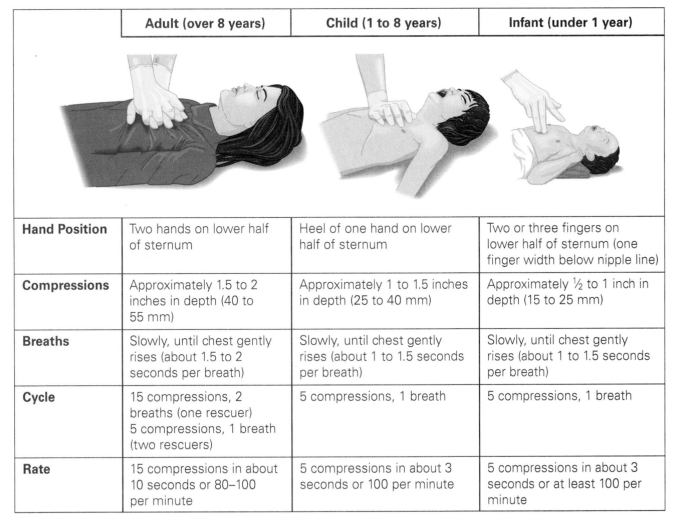

	Adult (over 8 years)	Child (1 to 8 years)	Infant (under 1 year)
Hand Position	Two hands on lower half of sternum	Heel of one hand on lower half of sternum	Two or three fingers on lower half of sternum (one finger width below nipple line)
Compressions	Approximately 1.5 to 2 inches in depth (40 to 55 mm)	Approximately 1 to 1.5 inches in depth (25 to 40 mm)	Approximately ½ to 1 inch in depth (15 to 25 mm)
Breaths	Slowly, until chest gently rises (about 1.5 to 2 seconds per breath)	Slowly, until chest gently rises (about 1 to 1.5 seconds per breath)	Slowly, until chest gently rises (about 1 to 1.5 seconds per breath)
Cycle	15 compressions, 2 breaths (one rescuer) 5 compressions, 1 breath (two rescuers)	5 compressions, 1 breath	5 compressions, 1 breath
Rate	15 compressions in about 10 seconds or 80–100 per minute	5 compressions in about 3 seconds or 100 per minute	5 compressions in about 3 seconds or at least 100 per minute

Figure 2-4 CPR Summary.

You could lose proper positioning. Avoid sudden jerky movements.

10. **Count as you administer compressions.** You should be able to say (and do) the following in a bit less than two seconds:

- One — push down.
- and — let up.
- Two — push down.
- and — let up.

This procedure should let you administer 80 to 100 compressions per minute to an adult. Practice until you can perform 15 complete compressions in 9 to 11 seconds. Beware of becoming hyperventilated. If you find you are, continue breathing at a regular tempo, but not at the same rhythm you used before.

One-Rescuer Adult CPR

To perform CPR alone, you must do the following: Determine unresponsiveness. Activate the EMS system, if it has not already been done. Open the airway, and determine breathlessness. Perform artificial ventilation, and remove foreign body airway obstructions as needed. If breathing is restored and the patient has a pulse, then place him or her in the recovery position. Do not begin CPR.

If the patient's pulse is absent, begin CPR as follows (Figure 2-7). Be certain that you have taken all proper BSI precautions. Then:

1. **Get in position,** and locate the proper hand position (described earlier).

2. **Perform chest compressions.** Perform 15 chest compressions at a rate of 80 to 100 per

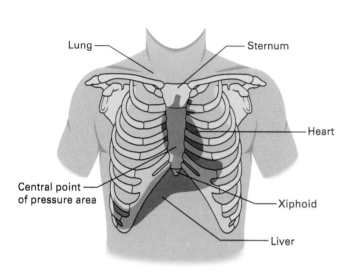

Lung — — Sternum

— Heart

Central point — of pressure area

— Xiphoid

— Liver

Posterior movement of xiphoid may lacerate liver. Lowest point of pressure on sternum must be above, not on, the xiphoid.

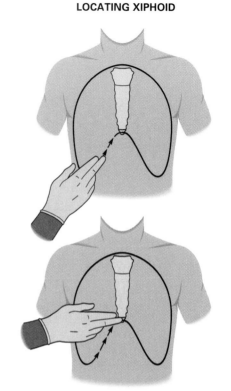

Figure 2-5   Locating the xiphoid process.

minute. Either count out loud or use some other way to keep track of the number of compressions you deliver.

3. **Deliver two slow breaths.** After completing 15 compressions, open the airway. Then deliver two breaths, each lasting 1.5 to 2 seconds. Be sure you inhale deeply between breaths. Continue until you have completed four cycles of 15 compressions and 2 ventilations.

4. **Then check the patient's pulse.** Check for 5 to 10 seconds at the carotid artery. If the pulse has returned, monitor the patient's pulse and breathing closely until the EMTs arrive. If the pulse has returned but the patient is not breathing, provide artificial ventilation. If there is still no pulse, resume CPR. Check again for pulse and breathing every two or three minutes.

If another First Responder trained in CPR arrives at the scene, he or she should do two things. First, the rescuer should verify that the EMS system has been activated and is responding. He should activate the EMS system, if necessary.

Second, the rescuer may take over CPR when the first rescuer gets tired.

To relieve the first rescuer with as little interruption as possible, follow these steps:

◆ If the first rescuer is currently performing chest compressions, the second rescuer should take a position at the patient's head. The second rescuer may then attempt to check the pulse while the first rescuer compresses the chest. Adequate CPR will usually create a carotid pulse. When the first rescuer completes the compressions, the second rescuer should provide two ventilations and check the pulse. The second rescuer can then resume CPR.

◆ If the first rescuer is performing ventilations when the second rescuer arrives, the second rescuer should prepare to perform compressions. After the first rescuer completes two ventilations and checks the pulse, the second rescuer should begin compressions.

There is no exact sequence to cover all situations. The examples above are efficient ways to change rescuers when performing CPR. The main

Correct Position for CPR

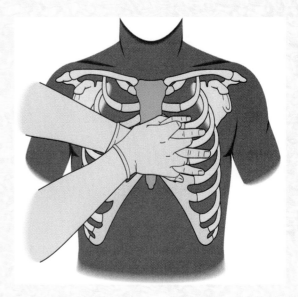

Figure 2-6a Place the heel of your hand on the patient's sternum.

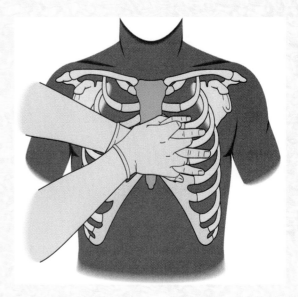

Figure 2-6b Interlace your fingers.

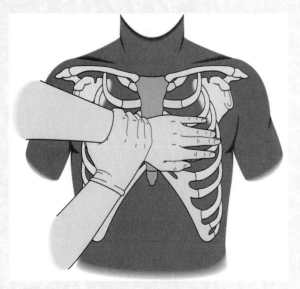

Figure 2-6c Alternative hand placement for large hands and hands or wrists with arthritis.

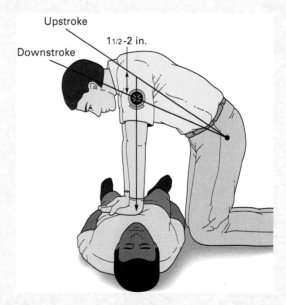

Upstroke

Downstroke

1 1/2 - 2 in.

Figure 2-6d Position your shoulders, and then perform chest compressions.

objective is to minimize the amount of time the patient goes without CPR. It is usually convenient to incorporate pulse and breathing checks into the changes.

Any rescuers who are not currently performing CPR can help prepare the scene for the arrival of the ambulance. EMTs and paramedics require space for stretchers, equipment, and additional personnel. Moving furniture away from the patient may help to create extra space. Directing the ambulance crew to the patient is also valuable. If time permits, find out from family and bystanders the exact sequence of events leading to the time the patient's heart stopped.

One-Rescuer Adult CPR

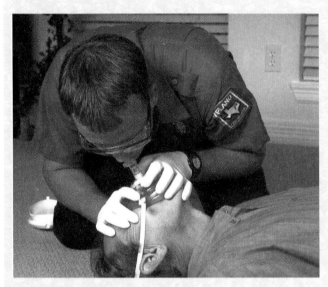

Figure 2-7a After determining unresponsiveness and breathlessness, provide artificial ventilation.

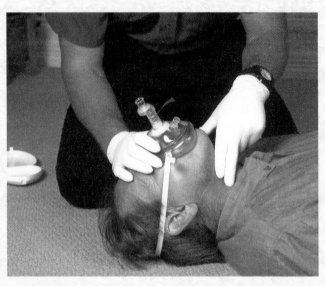

Figure 2-7b Determine pulselessness.

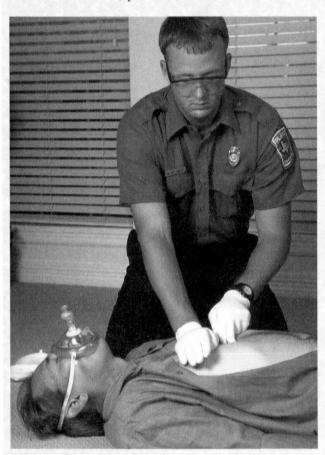

Figure 2-7c Expose chest, and locate proper hand position.

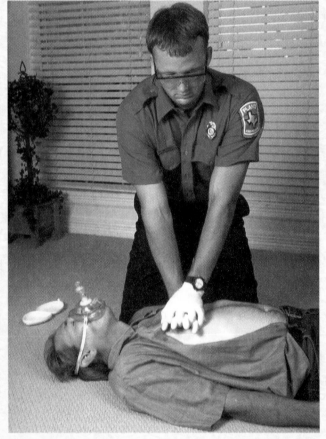

Figure 2-7d Perform chest compressions and ventilations at the proper rate.

Two-Rescuer Adult CPR

All First Responders should learn both the one-rescuer and two-rescuer techniques. The two-rescuer coordinated technique is less tiring. When possible, use an oral airway and a pocket face mask.

Before performing CPR, you and your partner must first determine that the patient is unresponsive, breathless, and pulseless. One rescuer may determine unresponsiveness, provide initial ventilations, and check the pulse. At the same time, the second rescuer can activate the EMS system and prepare to do compressions.

Note that in two-rescuer CPR, the ratio of compressions to ventilations is 5:1 (five compressions and then one ventilation). The ventilation should be delivered during a 1.5- to 2-second pause after every fifth chest compression.

If the patient remains unresponsive, breathless, and pulseless after your initial breaths, proceed as follows (Figure 2-8):

1. **Get in position.** The rescuers, if possible, should take position on opposite sides of the patient. One rescuer kneels by the patient's side for compressions. The other kneels at the patient's head and provides ventilations.

2. **Perform five chest compressions.** Perform them at a rate of 80 to 100 per minute. The compression rescuer should count the sequence out loud. Use an audible count of "one and two and three and four and five and pause," so that five compressions can be achieved every three to five seconds.

3. **Deliver one slow breath.** The ventilation rescuer should take a deep breath on "three and," get into position to ventilate on "four and," and begin breathing into the patient after "five." The compression rescuer pauses for 1.5 to 2 seconds so that the patient receives a slow, full breath. If you have the proper equipment and training, ventilate with 100% oxygen.

4. **After one minute of CPR, check the patient's pulse.** Check for 5 to 10 seconds at the carotid artery. If the pulse has returned, monitor the patient's pulse and breathing closely until the EMTs arrive. If the pulse has returned but the patient is not breathing, provide artificial ventilation. If there is still no pulse, resume CPR. Check again for pulse and breathing every two or three minutes.

When the compression rescuer gets tired, he or she should switch with the ventilation rescuer. Here is the seven-second method (Figure 2-9):

1. The tired compression rescuer calls for a switch at the beginning of the compression cycle by substituting "change" for "one." The audible count remains the same for the remaining four compressions. (Any mnemonic that satisfactorily accomplishes the change is acceptable. Another popular technique uses "Change, on, the, next, breath.") A similar phrase can also be used to call for the move of the patient or for a pulse check. It simply involves substituting. For example:

   ◆ "1 and 2 and 3 and 4 and 5 and pause."
   ◆ "Change and 2 and 3 and 4 and 5 and pause."
   ◆ "Lift and 2 and 3 and 4 and 5 and pause."
   ◆ "Pulse and 2 and 3 and 4 and 5 and pause."

2. After the fifth compression, the ventilation rescuer should give a full breath. Then he or she should move to the chest, locate the xiphoid process, and get hands in position for compressions.

3. At the same time, the compression rescuer should move quickly to the patient's head. Then he or she checks the carotid pulse and breathing for three to five seconds.

4. If no pulse is found, the rescuer at the head gives a breath and announces, "No pulse. Continue CPR."

5. The rescuer at the chest is in position and begins compression. If shortness of breath prevents the rescuer from giving a full count out loud, he or she should at least say the "four and five and" count so that the ventilation rescuer will know when to breathe.

Monitoring the Patient

The patient's condition needs to be monitored throughout CPR. This will ensure that rescue efforts are effective. It also lets you know when spontaneous breathing and the pulse returns.

In two-rescuer CPR, there is a ventilation rescuer and a compression rescuer. To monitor the effectiveness of chest compressions, the ventilation rescuer should feel for a pulse at the carotid artery during compressions. To determine if a spontaneous pulse has returned, the ventilation rescuer should check the carotid artery for three

Two-Rescuer Adult CPR

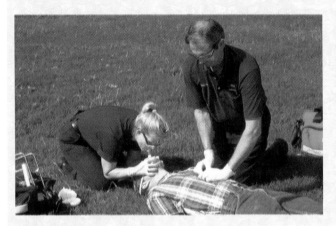

Figure 2-8a The ventilation rescuer provides artificial ventilation while the compression rescuer bares the patient's chest.

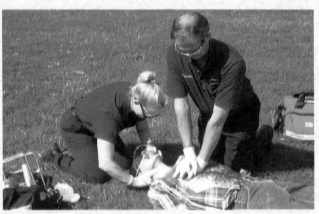

Figure 2-8b The ventilation rescuer determines pulselessness as the compression rescuer gets into position.

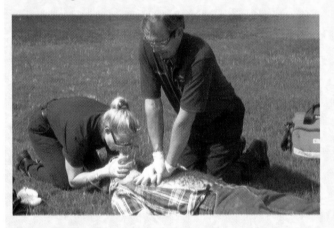

Figure 2-8c Both work together to perform compressions and ventilations at the correct ratio and rate.

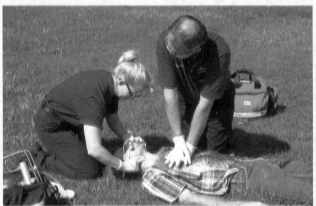

Figure 2-8d After the first minute and every few minutes thereafter, stop CPR to assess the carotid pulse.

to five seconds at the end of the first minute of CPR and every few minutes thereafter. Note that the pulse must be checked when CPR is not in progress.

In general, CPR should not be interrupted for more than five seconds. One of the few exceptions to this rule applies to moving a patient. It may not be possible to perform CPR in a cramped bedroom or other small area. In this case, it is acceptable to move the patient so proper CPR can be performed. These actions must be kept as close to five seconds as possible.

Signs of Successful CPR

Signs of successful CPR include the following:

◆ Each time the sternum is compressed, you should feel a pulse in the carotid artery. It may feel like a flutter.

◆ Chest should rise and fall with each ventilation.

◆ Patient's skin color may improve or return to normal.

Other possible but less likely occurrences include:

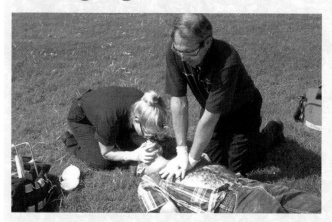

Figure 2-9a The tired compression rescuer calls for a switch.

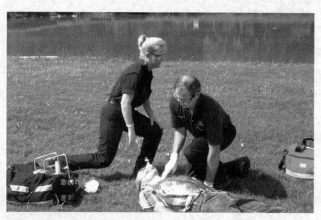

Figure 2-9b The ventilation rescuer delivers a breath as usual, then moves to the patient's side. The second rescuer moves to the patient's head.

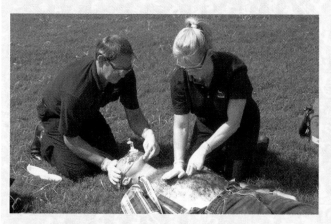

Figure 2-9c The rescuer at the head opens the airway and checks respirations and pulse for five seconds. The second rescuer prepares for compressions.

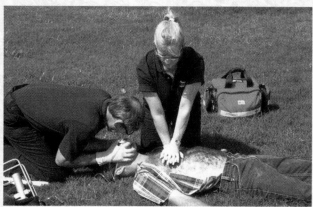

Figure 2-9d If the patient is still unresponsive, breathless, and pulseless, continue CPR.

◆ Pupils may react or appear to be normal. (Pupils should constrict when exposed to light.)

◆ Heartbeat may return.

◆ Spontaneous gasp of breathing may occur.

◆ Patient may move his or her own arms or legs.

◆ Patient may try to swallow.

Remember that "successful" CPR does not mean that the patient lives. "Successful" only means that you performed CPR correctly. Very few patients will survive if they do not receive early defibrillation and advanced cardiac life support (ACLS). The goal of CPR is to extend the window of survival. Hopefully, advanced providers will arrive in time.

Mistakes in Performing CPR

The most common ventilation mistakes are as follows:

◆ Failing to maintain an adequate head tilt.

◆ Failing to maintain an adequate seal around the patient's mouth, nose, or both with a pocket face mask or face shield. The seal should be released when the patient exhales.

- Completing a two-rescuer cycle in fewer than five seconds.
- Failing to watch and listen for exhalation.
- Not giving full breaths.
- Providing breaths too rapidly.

Some common chest compression mistakes include the following:

- Bending your elbows instead of keeping them straight.
- Not aligning your shoulders directly above the patient's sternum.
- Placing the heel of your bottom hand too low or not in line with the sternum (Figure 2-10).
- Not depressing the sternum to proper depth.
- Not extending the fingers of your hands, touching the patient's chest.
- Pivoting at the knees instead of at your hips.
- Compressing at an incorrect rate.
- Moving your hands from the compression site between compressions.

Complications Caused by CPR

Even properly performed, CPR may cause rib fractures in some patients. Other complications that can occur with proper CPR include:

- Fracture of the sternum, which is common in older patients.
- Pneumothorax (collapse of the lungs caused by air in the chest).

- Hemothorax (collapse of the lungs caused by bleeding in the chest).
- Cuts and bruises to the lungs.
- Lacerations (cuts) to the liver.

These complications are rare. However, you can help minimize the risk by giving careful attention to your performance. Remember that effective CPR is necessary, even if it results in complications. After all, the alternative is death.

In addition, the rib cartilage in elderly patients separates easily. You will hear it crunch as you compress. Be sure that your hand is positioned correctly and that you are compressing to the correct depth, but do not stop.

CPR for Infants and Children

Infants (up to one year old) and children (one to eight years old) need slightly different care. Cardiac arrest in them is rarely caused by heart problems. The heart nearly always stops beating because of too little oxygen due to injuries, suffocation, smoke inhalation, **sudden infant death syndrome (SIDS),** or infection.

Remember that according to AHA guidelines, if you are alone, you should resuscitate an infant or child for one minute before you activate the EMS system.

Determining that your infant or child patient is pulseless is important. For an infant, check the brachial pulse on the inside of the upper arm between the elbow and shoulder. Press the artery gently with your index and middle fingers. Never use your thumb. In a child, check the pulse at the carotid artery.

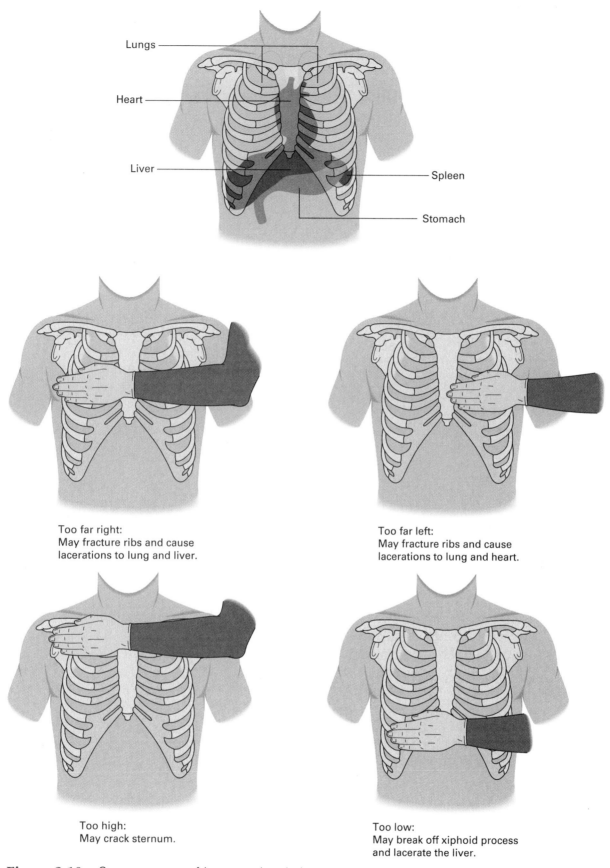

Too far right:
May fracture ribs and cause lacerations to lung and liver.

Too far left:
May fracture ribs and cause lacerations to lung and heart.

Too high:
May crack sternum.

Too low:
May break off xiphoid process and lacerate the liver.

Figure 2-10 Consequences of improper hand placement.

Infant and Child CPR

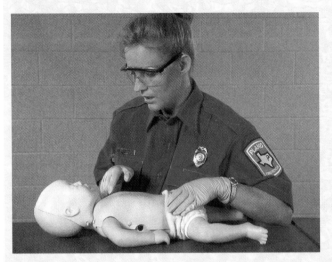

Figure 2-11a Determine unresponsiveness by tapping the infant and speaking loudly.

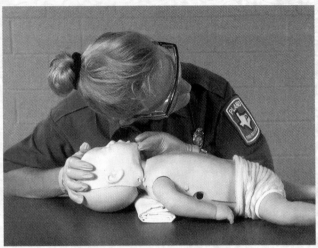

Figure 2-11b Gently open the airway, and determine breathlessness.

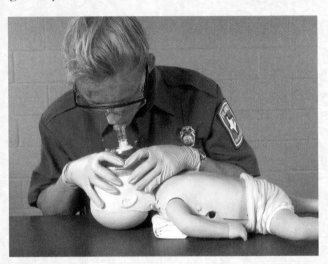

Figure 2-11c Cover the infant's mouth and nose with a pocket mask. Then ventilate.

It can be difficult to find a pulse in an infant or child. *So, do not spend too much time trying to locate one.* According to the AHA, if the infant or child is not breathing, heart rate is probably inadequate and chest compressions are usually necessary.

Performing Infant or Child CPR

If the infant or child is unresponsive, breathless, and pulseless, begin CPR. Be certain you have

taken BSI precautions. Then follow these guidelines (Figures 2-11 and 2-12):

1. **Position the patient.** Make sure the patient is lying on a firm, flat surface. If the patient is an infant, put him or her in your lap with head tilted back slightly. Use your palm to support the baby's back. Make sure his or her head is not higher than the rest of the body.

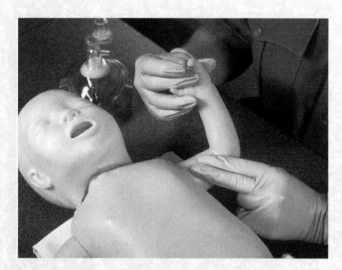

Figure 2-11d Determine pulselessness at the brachial artery.

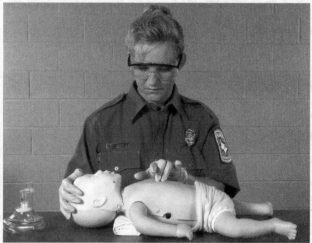

Figure 2-11e Locate the correct hand position, and begin chest compressions.

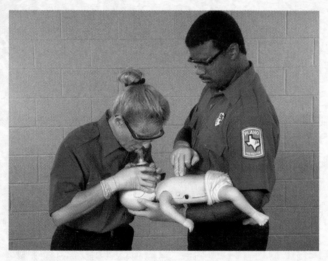

Figure 2-11f Performing CPR while carrying the baby.

2. **Locate the compression site.** For an infant, it is one finger-width below an imaginary line between the nipples.

   For a child, locate the lower margin of the rib cage on the side next to you. Use your middle and index fingers, while your hand nearest the child's head maintains head tilt. Follow the rib cage to the xiphoid process, where the ribs and sternum meet. Then place your index finger next to the middle finger.

While looking at the position of the index finger, lift that hand and place its heel next to where the index finger was.

3. **Perform chest compressions.** For an infant, use the flat part of your middle and ring fingers to compress the infant's sternum one-half to one inch (15 mm to 25 mm), or one-third to one-half of the depth of the chest. The compression rate for an infant is at least 100 per minute.

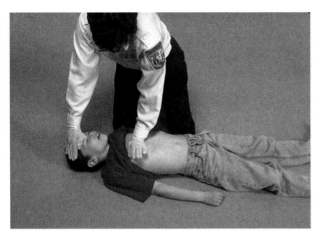

Figure 2-12 Chest compressions on a larger child.

For a child, compress the sternum 1.0 inch to 1.5 inches (25 mm to 40 mm), or one-third to one-half of the depth of the chest, with the heel of one hand. The compression rate for a child is 100 compressions per minute.

The ratio of compressions to ventilations in both infants and children is 5:1 (five compressions and then one ventilation). In one-rescuer CPR for an infant or child, ventilate during a pause after each fifth compression. Count compressions at this rhythm:

◆ Infant—1, 2, 3, 4, 5, breathe.
◆ Child—1 and 2 and 3 and 4 and 5 and breathe.

After one minute, or 20 cycles, check for the return of a spontaneous pulse.

Signs of Successful Infant and Child CPR

The methods of checking for successful CPR in infants and children are almost the same as for adults.

◆ Check the patient's pulse periodically. In the infant, check the brachial pulse. In the child, check the carotid pulse.
◆ Check the pupils. CPR is successful if they are reacting normally or appear to be normal.
◆ Watch for a spontaneous heartbeat, spontaneous breathing, and responsiveness.

Complications of Infant and Child CPR

One of the most common complications with injury and sudden illness in children is hypothermia (a below-normal body temperature). So keep the infant or child warm.

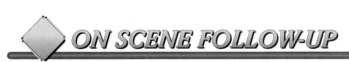

ON SCENE FOLLOW-UP

At the beginning of this chapter, you read that First Responders took over CPR from a bystander. To see how chapter skills apply to this emergency, read the following. It describes how the call was completed.

PHYSICAL EXAMINATION

Our first concern was providing good CPR. Two rescuers in my crew were doing that. A thorough physical exam would have to wait. The patient was on the living room floor and didn't appear to have any injuries from falling to the ground.

PATIENT HISTORY

I talked to the bystander who had identified himself earlier as the patient's brother. He told me that the patient had been mowing the lawn when he began having chest pain. He stated that his brother had entered the living room, clutching his chest and complaining of pressure beneath his breast bone. A minute later, he witnessed the collapse to the floor. He stated he thought the patient had collapsed about five minutes before we arrived.

The patient's wife was also in the house. She told me that her husband was 71 and had bypass surgery two years ago after a heart attack. He was on medication for his heart and high blood pressure. She went to get it, as I radioed the incoming EMS units with an update.

ONGOING ASSESSMENT

I assumed the role of "safety officer" and monitored the effectiveness of the ongoing CPR. I also maintained contact with the responding ambulance crew. I asked my crew members if either of them needed a break. They stated they were okay. All we could do at this point was await the EMT's arrival. It seemed like it took them forever, yet within four minutes they were on scene.

PATIENT HAND-OFF

When the EMTs arrived, I told them that the patient is a 71-year-old male. He was mowing the lawn and then entered the house complaining of chest pain. He collapsed to the floor while talking to his brother. While his brother called 9-1-1, the wife began CPR. The patient was unresponsive with no pulse or respirations when CPR was continued by our crew. I told them I didn't believe the patient had any injuries. He had a history of bypass surgery and high blood pressure, and took medication. I gave them the patient's medication vials.

The EMTs continued emergency care as we watched. It took three shocks from the AED to get the patient's heart started again. But he still had no respirations. So one of them continued to ventilate the patient while the others put the patient on a backboard. The backboard would give them a hard surface to compress against in case they had to start CPR again.

Later, the EMTs told me that the patient had improved slightly in the ambulance and was transferred to the cardiac unit at the hospital. Not all patients survive. I was happy we helped one who did.

Heart disease is still the number one killer in the U.S. Be prepared to provide CPR to any patient who needs it, and remember to take refresher courses frequently.

Chapter Review

Circulation, like respiration, is essential to life. If a patient's heart fails to beat, he or she will surely die unless actions are taken to restore the heartbeat. As a First Responder, you will help to take these actions.

Cardiopulmonary resuscitation (CPR) is the first step in saving the life of a patient whose heart has stopped beating. The sooner CPR is started, the better, because permanent brain damage may occur after as few as four minutes.

The AED is a device that applies an electric shock to the patient's chest, which can restore a heartbeat. You will recall that the chain of survival requires early access, early CPR, and early defibrillation together with advanced care for an optimal chance of survival.

Perform CPR in accordance with AHA standards when you are called to do so. Be sure you have a barrier device with you at all times.

FIRE COMPANY REVIEW

Page references where answers may be found or supported are provided at the end of each question.

Section 1

1. What is the name and location of each of the four chambers of the heart? (p. 25)
2. What are the links in the "chain of survival"? (pp. 26–27)
3. What is the pulse? Where can you best palpate it? (pp. 25–26)

Section 2

4. Before performing CPR on your patient, what must your assessment of his or her condition reveal? (p. 27)

5. How can you find the correct CPR compression site on an infant, child, and adult? (pp. 29, 41)
6. What are the appropriate compression depths for an infant, child, and adult? (pp. 30, 41–42)
7. Why is it essential to perform CPR in spite of the problems it may cause? (p. 38)
8. When should you activate EMS if your patient is an unresponsive adult? An unresponsive infant? (pp. 27, 38)

RESOURCES TO LEARN MORE

Basic Life Support for Healthcare Providers: 1997–99 Emergency Cardiovascular Care Programs. Dallas: American Heart Association, 1997.

Heartsaver Plus: 1997–99 Emergency Cardiovascular Care Programs. Dallas: American Heart Association, 1997.

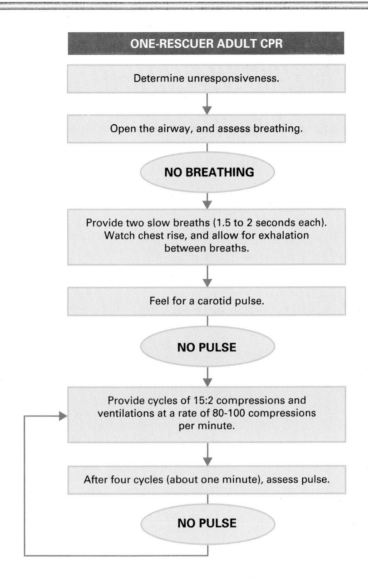

ONE-RESCUER ADULT CPR

Determine unresponsiveness.

Open the airway, and assess breathing.

NO BREATHING

Provide two slow breaths (1.5 to 2 seconds each). Watch chest rise, and allow for exhalation between breaths.

Feel for a carotid pulse.

NO PULSE

Provide cycles of 15:2 compressions and ventilations at a rate of 80-100 compressions per minute.

After four cycles (about one minute), assess pulse.

NO PULSE

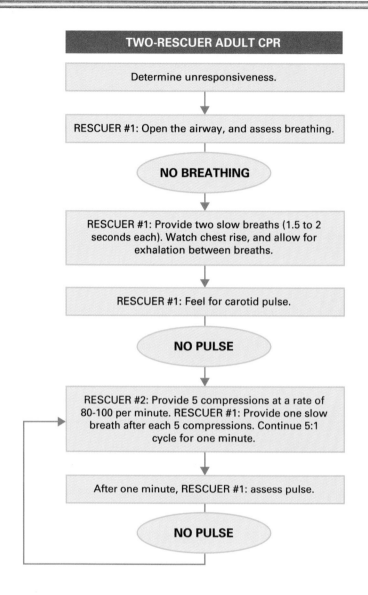

TWO-RESCUER ADULT CPR

Determine unresponsiveness.

RESCUER #1: Open the airway, and assess breathing.

NO BREATHING

RESCUER #1: Provide two slow breaths (1.5 to 2 seconds each). Watch chest rise, and allow for exhalation between breaths.

RESCUER #1: Feel for carotid pulse.

NO PULSE

RESCUER #2: Provide 5 compressions at a rate of 80-100 per minute. RESCUER #1: Provide one slow breath after each 5 compressions. Continue 5:1 cycle for one minute.

After one minute, RESCUER #1: assess pulse.

NO PULSE

Bleeding and Shock

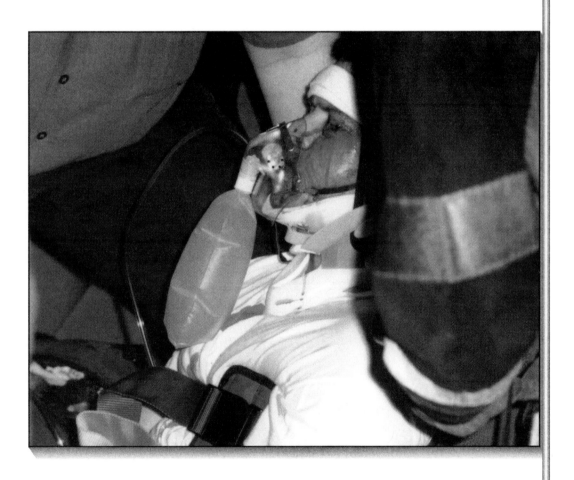

*I*NTRODUCTION   *Any unchecked bleeding can create a life-threatening situation for your patient. It does not really matter if it is visible (external) or invisible (internal) bleeding. Before the patient dies, however, the phenomena known as "shock" occurs. What is shock? It is defined as a lack of tissue **perfusion**. This inability of the body to deliver oxygenated blood to the cells, or **hypoperfusion,** has characteristics that are clearly identifiable by the well-trained fire service First Responder. Early recognition of the signs and symptoms of shock can allow you to deliver quick, life-saving treatment to your patient.*

Cognitive, affective, and psychomotor objectives are from the U.S. DOT's "First Responder: National Standard Curriculum." Enrichment objectives, if any, identify supplemental material.

Cognitive

5-2.1 Differentiate between arterial, venous, and capillary bleeding. (p. 50)

5-2.2 State the emergency medical care for external bleeding. (pp. 50, 52–55)

5-2.3 Establish the relationship between body substance isolation and bleeding. (p. 49)

5-2.4 List the signs of internal bleeding. (pp. 55–56)

5-2.5 List the steps in the emergency medical care of the patient with signs and symptoms of internal bleeding. (p. 56)

Affective

5-2.15 Explain the rationale for body substance isolation when dealing with bleeding and soft tissue injuries. (p. 49)

5-2.16 Attend to the feelings of the patient with a soft tissue injury or bleeding. (pp. 52–53)

5-2.17 Demonstrate a caring attitude towards patients with a soft tissue injury or bleeding who request emergency medical services. (pp. 52–53)

5-2.18 Place the interests of the patient with a soft tissue injury or bleeding as the foremost consideration when making any and all patient care decisions. (pp. 50, 52–53)

5-2.19 Communicate with empathy to patients with a soft tissue injury or bleeding, as well as with family members and friends of the patient. (p. 53)

Psychomotor

5-2.20 Demonstrate direct pressure as a method of emergency medical care for external bleeding. (p. 52)

5-2.21 Demonstrate the use of diffuse pressure as a method of emergency medical care for external bleeding. (p. 52)

5-2.22 Demonstrate the use of pressure points as a method of emergency medical care for external bleeding. (p. 52)

5-2.23 Demonstrate the care of the patient exhibiting signs and symptoms of internal bleeding. (p. 56)

Enrichment

◆ Discuss the use of splints and tourniquets as methods of bleeding control. (pp. 53–54)

◆ Describe emergency care of a patient with a nosebleed. (pp. 54–55)

◆ List the causes of shock. (p. 56)

◆ Describe the compensatory, decompensated, and irreversible stages of shock. (pp. 56–58)

◆ Describe the emergency care of a patient in shock. (pp. 58–59, 61)

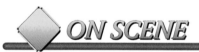 ON SCENE

DISPATCH

While training outside the fire station, the engine company was dispatched for a fall injury. Since we had been practicing hose evolutions, most of us were already in our turnout gear. En route, we were notified by dispatch that a 41-year-old male had fallen from his roof while removing holiday lights.

SCENE SIZE-UP

Before arriving on scene, all responders had taken BSI precautions. Upon arrival, we encountered a woman kneeling beside a person who was supine in the front yard. The woman got up and approached us. She identified herself as the patient's spouse and stated that her husband, Dan Williams, had fallen from the roof but was conscious. We noted that the fall was about 18 to 20 feet (6 m to 7 m) onto a grassy lawn.

INITIAL ASSESSMENT

My general impression revealed a conscious male patient, whose eyes were open and who was talking coherently. I observed his breathing, which appeared to be a little too fast. There were no obvious signs of external bleeding.

As I introduced myself to the patient, another member of our engine company provided manual stabilization of the patient's head and neck. I assessed a radial pulse, which was rapid. I also noted that the patient's skin was cool and clammy despite the 80°F (27°C) air temperature. I then asked one of my partners to administer oxygen via a nonrebreather mask at a flow rate of 15 liters per minute.

PHYSICAL EXAMINATION

Dan complained that his stomach hurt. When I asked what happened, he stated he was removing holiday lights from his roof when he slipped and fell face first onto the ground. He said he hadn't lost consciousness. He stated he was thirsty and asked if we could get him a drink of water. I informed him that we could not allow him to drink anything at this time. Dan then became upset with us, and wondered aloud why we didn't "leave him alone."

I explained to Dan that we were there to help him, and asked if I might remove his shirt to further assess his condition. He gave us permission, and I began assessing his chest and abdomen. When I gently palpated the left upper abdominal quadrant, I noticed it was unusually hard—more so than the right. Dan also winced in pain while I did this, stating that his stomach was "really sore." At this point, I asked my partner to contact the ambulance and determine their ETA.

Dan's baseline vital signs were pulse 124, blood pressure 130/70, and respirations 28.

PATIENT HISTORY

Dan was 41 years old, and he told us he had no medical conditions. I asked if he was taking any medications or was allergic to anything. He stated he was taking ibuprofen for an arthritic knee, and was not allergic to anything. I told Dan I was going to give him a number to remember: the number 51. I asked if he would repeat it and he said "the number is 51." I also explained to Dan why we were doing this.

As you read the following chapter, consider these questions: Is this patient bleeding? Is this patient in shock? How would you treat him?

BLEEDING

Body Substance Isolation (BSI)

Always take BSI precautions to protect against diseases transmitted by way of blood and body fluids. This is especially true when the patient is bleeding. You should:

◆ Keep a barrier between you and the patient's blood and body fluids. Wear the appropriate protective equipment, such as gloves and eyewear.

◆ Never touch your nose, mouth, or eyes or handle food while providing emergency care.

◆ Keep all of the patient's open wounds—*and all of yours*—covered with dressings or sterile bandages.

◆ Wash your hands properly as soon as possible after treating a patient.

If any equipment, turnout gear, helmets, and so on have been exposed to a patient's blood or body fluids, they must be cleaned as soon as possible. Follow your local disinfecting protocol.

How the Body Responds to Blood Loss

Blood is the fluid component of the circulatory system (Figure 3-1). One of its critical functions is the transport of oxygen to cells. This is called **perfusion.** After unloading its cargo of oxygen, blood then transports the waste product of

DISTRIBUTION OF BLOOD
IN THE BODY

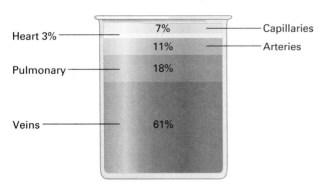

Heart 3% ——— 7% ——— Capillaries
              11% ——— Arteries
Pulmonary ——— 18%

Veins ——— 61%

Figure 3-1   Blood is part of the circulatory system.

cells—carbon dioxide—back to the lungs. This process can be impaired by as little as one liter (1000 cc) of sudden blood loss in an adult, and as little as one-half liter (500 cc) in a child. Left unchecked, death may result. (See Figure 3-2.)

External Bleeding

External bleeding occurs from three types of blood vessels: arteries, veins, and capillaries. Bleeding from any of these vessels can be life-threatening if not properly treated. Each type of bleeding has its own unique characteristics (Figure 3-3):

◆ *Arterial bleeding.* Bright red blood spurting from an open wound usually indicates a damaged or severed artery. The blood is a bright red color because it is rich in oxygen. Since arteries are "high pressure" vessels, this type of bleeding can be difficult to control.

◆ *Venous bleeding.* This is usually a darker red color than arterial blood. This type of bleeding is characterized by a slow, yet steady flow. The blood is a darker red color because it has little, if any, oxygen. The flow is steady,

because veins are "low pressure" vessels. Venous bleeding is usually easier to control than arterial bleeding.

◆ *Capillary bleeding.* This is the most common type of bleeding encountered with injured patients. It is characterized by oozing, dark red blood. Because capillaries are tiny "low pressure" vessels, this type of bleeding is usually easily controlled.

◆ *Emergency Care*

All external bleeding must be controlled as soon as possible during the initial assessment. Although airway and breathing take precedence, in most instances bleeding control will occur at the same time that airway and breathing are being managed.

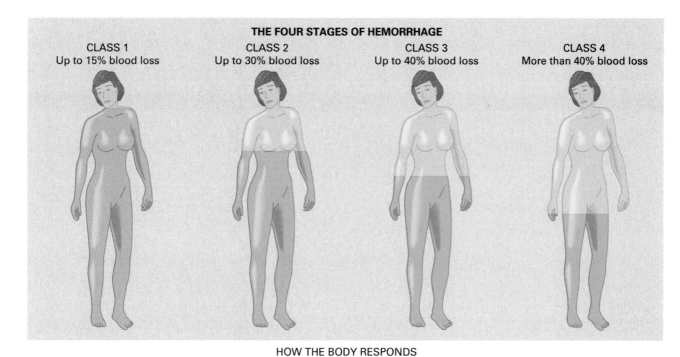

THE FOUR STAGES OF HEMORRHAGE

CLASS 1	CLASS 2	CLASS 3	CLASS 4
Up to 15% blood loss	Up to 30% blood loss	Up to 40% blood loss	More than 40% blood loss

HOW THE BODY RESPONDS

The body compensates for blood loss by constricting blood vessels (vasoconstriction) in an effort to maintain blood pressure and delivery of oxygen to all organs of the body.

EFFECT ON PATIENT

• Patient remains alert.
• Blood pressure stays within normal limits.
• Pulse stays within normal limits or increases slightly; pulse quality remains strong.
• Respiratory rate and depth, skin color and temperature all remain normal.

*The average adult has 5 liters (1 liter = approximately 1 quart) of circulating blood; 15% is 750 ml (or about 3 cups). With internal bleeding 750 ml will occupy enough space in a limb to cause swelling and pain. With bleeding into the body cavities, however, the blood will spread throughout the cavity, causing little, if any initial discomfort.

• Vasoconstriction continues to maintain adequate blood pressure, but with some difficulty now.
• Blood flow is shunted to vital organs, with decreased flow to intestines, kidneys, and skin.

EFFECT ON PATIENT

• Patient may become confused and restless.
• Skin turns pale, cool, and dry because of shunting of blood to vital organs.
• Diastolic pressure may rise or fall. It's more likely to rise (because of vasoconstriction) or stay the same in otherwise healthy patients with no underlying cardio-vascular problems.
• Pulse pressure (difference between systolic and diastolic pressures) narrows.
• Sympathetic responses also cause rapid heart rate (over 100 beats per minute). Pulse quality weakens.
• Respiratory rate increases because of sympathetic stimulation.
• Delayed capillary refill.

• Compensatory mechanisms become overtaxed. Vaso-constriction, for example, can no longer sustain blood pressure, which now begins to fall.
• Cardiac output and tissue perfusion continue to decrease, becoming potentially life threatening. (Even at this stage, however, the patient can still recover with prompt treatment.)

EFFECT ON PATIENT

• Patient becomes more confused, restless, and anxious.
• Classic signs of shock appear—rapid heart rate, decreased blood pressure, rapid respiration and cool, clammy extremities.

• Compensatory vasoconstriction now becomes a complicating factor in itself, further impairing tissue perfusion and cellular oxygenation.

EFFECT ON PATIENT

• Patient becomes lethargic, drowsy, or stuporous.
• Signs of shock become more pronounced. Blood pressure continues to fall.
• Lack of blood flow to the brain and other vital organs ultimately leads to organ failure and death.

Figure 3-2   Four stages of hemorrhage.

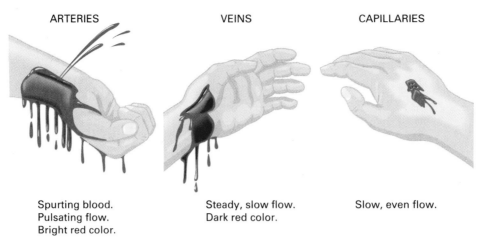

ARTERIES   VEINS   CAPILLARIES

Spurting blood.
Pulsating flow.
Bright red color.

Steady, slow flow.
Dark red color.

Slow, even flow.

Figure 3-3   Types of external bleeding.

There are four basic methods of controlling external bleeding. They can be recalled by the mnemonic **DEPS:**

D — Direct pressure.
E — Elevation.
P — Pressure points.
S — Splinting.

For a patient with external bleeding, take BSI precautions and follow these steps (Figure 3-4):

1. **Apply direct pressure to the wound.** Direct pressure will stop blood from flowing into the damaged vessel, helping it to clot. Do this by placing a gloved hand over the wound until a sterile dressing can be applied. If the wound is small, apply pressure directly over it with your fingertips. If the wound is large, the flat part of your hand may be necessary to control the bleeding. Large gaping wounds may require sterile gauze and direct hand pressure if fingertip pressure fails to control bleeding.

   One effective way to maintain direct pressure over a wound on an extremity is through the use of an air splint. Apply it directly on top of the wound (Figure 3-5).

2. **Elevate the bleeding extremity.** Do this at the same time you are applying direct pressure. Ideally, the limb should be elevated above the level of the heart. However, do not elevate it if you suspect a bone or joint injury.

3. **Assess bleeding.** After applying direct pressure and using elevation, assess the wound. If the bleeding has soaked through the dressing, apply another dressing on top of it.

4. **If bleeding is not yet controlled, use pressure points.** (See Figure 3-6.) For bleeding in the forearm, find the brachial pulse point, which overlies the upper arm. Using the flat surface of your fingers, compress the artery against the bone, slowing the flow of blood below that point.

   For bleeding in the leg, find the femoral pulse point. Then compress the artery against the pelvis using the heel of your hand.

🔔 **FIRE DRILL**

Your patients do not care how much you know until they know how much you care! Therefore, administer a large dose of reassurance as often as possible.

NOTE: In some EMS systems, bleeding control procedures are slightly different. After you find that direct pressure and elevation do not work to stop bleeding, in those systems you are required to remove the first dressing to assess the bleeding point. If it is still bleeding or if there is more than one bleeding point, then you are to apply more pressure directly to the point or points. If this still does not control bleeding, you are to use pressure points as described above. Removing the first dressing to assess the bleeding is a controversial technique. Be sure to follow your own local protocols.

Throughout emergency care, provide emotional support to your patient. The sight of an arm or leg

Methods of Bleeding Control

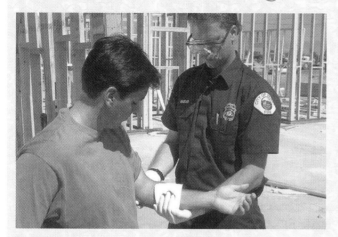

Figure 3-4a Apply direct pressure.

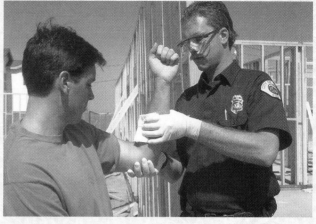

Figure 3-4b Elevate an extremity.

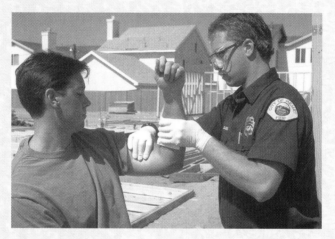

Figure 3-4c Use pressure points.

soaked in blood can be quite unnerving to anyone, young or old. Reassure your patient. Be honest, and communicate with empathy. Remember, staying calm throughout emergency care is a must.

Splinting

Splinting, or immobilization, is another way to control bleeding in an extremity. It works because movement promotes blood flow, which can disrupt the clotting process. So if a limb does not move, less blood reaches it and clotting is enhanced. Any splint will work. However, using an air splint can immobilize the limb as well as maintain direct pressure, which can free you up

for other duties. NOTE: It is probable that a combination of direct pressure, elevation, pressure points, and splinting will be used to control external bleeding.

Some EMS systems do not permit First Responders to splint, or immobilize, an injured limb. In many of those systems, manual stabilization of the limb is recommended instead. Always follow local protocol.

Tourniquets

A tourniquet should be used to control life-threatening bleeding when all other methods have failed. Because it can stop all blood flow to

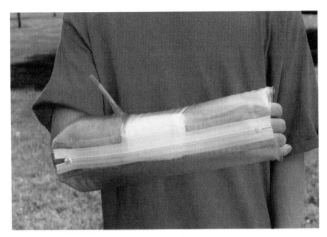

Figure 3-5 One way to maintain direct pressure is by use of an air splint.

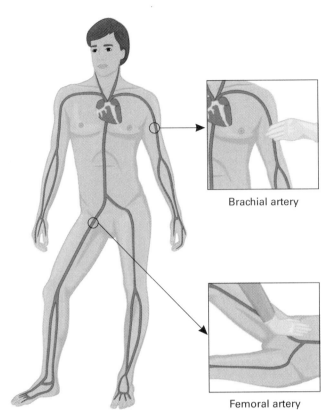

Figure 3-6 Pressure points in the extremities.

an extremity, use a tourniquet only as a last resort. A tourniquet can cause permanent damage to nerves, muscles, and blood vessels, and it can result in the loss of the affected limb. Always seek medical direction before using a tourniquet. Follow all local protocols. To apply a tourniquet:

1. **Select a bandage.** It should be 4 inches (100 mm) wide and six to eight layers deep.
2. **Wrap it around the extremity twice** at a point above but as close to the wound as possible.
3. **Tie a knot in the bandage material.** Then place a stick or rod on top of it. Tie the ends of the bandage again in a square knot over the stick.
4. **Twist the stick until the bleeding stops.** Then secure the stick or rod in place.
5. **Note the time.**
6. **Notify the EMTs** who take over patient care that you have applied a tourniquet.

In some cases an inflated blood pressure cuff may be used as a tourniquet until bleeding stops. If you choose to do this, you need to monitor the cuff continuously to make sure pressure is maintained.

When using any type of tourniquet, take the following precautions:

◆ Always use a wide bandage, and secure it tightly. Never use a wire, belt, or any other material that could cut the skin or underlying soft tissues.

◆ Once applied, never loosen or remove a tourniquet unless you are directed to do so by medical direction.

◆ Never apply a tourniquet directly over a joint.

◆ Always make sure the tourniquet is in open view. If it is covered by bandages or clothing, it may be overlooked, which can result in permanent tissue damage.

Nosebleeds

Causes of nosebleeds can range from injury, to disease, to the environment. Often more annoying than serious, nosebleeds also can be life-threatening. For example, nosebleeds associated with a fracture can be severe enough to compromise the airway and cause shock (hypoperfusion).

In most cases a nosebleed may be treated as follows (Figure 3-7):

Method of Nosebleed Control

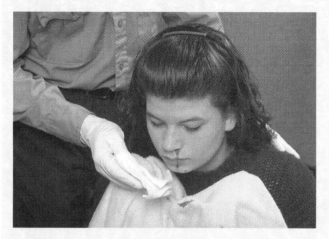

Figure 3-7a Keep the patient quiet and leaning forward in a sitting position.

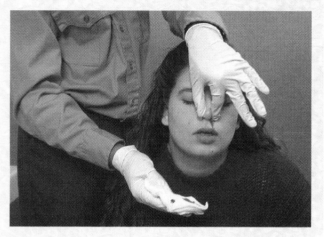

Figure 3-7b Apply pressure by pinching the nostrils. Also apply cold compresses if needed.

1. **Keep the patient calm.**
2. **Position the patient.** Have the patient sit and lean forward in order to prevent aspiration of blood into the lungs. If that is not possible, the patient should lie down with head and shoulders elevated. Be sure to maintain an open airway.
3. **Have the patient pinch the nostrils together,** if you do not suspect a broken nose.
4. **Slow the flow of blood.** Apply ice packs or cold compresses to the nose and face. Instruct the patient to avoid blowing his or her nose for several hours. It could dislodge the clot and restart bleeding.
5. **Activate the EMS system,** if bleeding continues and cannot be stopped.

If a fractured skull is suspected, do not try to stop a nosebleed. To do so might increase pressure on the brain. Instead, cover the nasal opening loosely with a dry, sterile dressing. Do not apply pressure. Treat the patient for a skull fracture.

Internal Bleeding

External bleeding is usually easy to spot. Internal bleeding is much more difficult to detect. This

GERIATRIC NOTE

A nosebleed in an elderly patient is often caused by severe hypertension. So, during scene size-up, look around the area. If you spot any medications, ask the patient what they are for. If there is reason to suspect hypertension, activate the EMS system. Hypertension could pose more of a problem than the nosebleed itself.

"invisible" blood loss can quickly result in death. So always maintain a high degree of suspicion whenever scrapes, bruises, swelling, deformity, or impact marks are present. Also assume internal bleeding with any penetrating wounds to the skull, chest, or abdomen.

The signs and symptoms of internal bleeding include:

◆ Pale, cool, clammy skin.
◆ Increased respiratory and pulse rates.
◆ Thirst.
◆ Changes in mental status, such as confusion, disorientation, and anxiety or agitation.
◆ Nausea and sometimes vomiting.
◆ Vomitus with blood.

- Dark, tarry stools.
- Discolored, tender, swollen, or hard tissue.
- Tender, rigid, or distended abdomen.
- Weakness, faintness, or dizziness.

◆ *Emergency Care*

When you suspect your patient is bleeding internally, immediately determine the ETA of the transporting unit. This patient needs rapid transport to a hospital. In the meantime, follow these steps:

1. **Establish and maintain an open airway.** If allowed, apply oxygen by way of a nonrebreather mask at 15 liters per minute. Ventilate, if necessary.

2. **Control external bleeding.** Since you cannot control internal bleeding, it becomes even more critical to control any external bleeding you observe.

3. **Keep your patient warm,** but take care to not overheat. Remember that a patient who loses a large amount of blood cannot conserve body heat effectively.

4. **Treat for shock.**

SECTION
2 SHOCK

To the lay person, shock can mean an unpleasant surprise or an electrical stimulus. For First Responders, however, shock (hypoperfusion) has a very precise definition. It is the inadequate delivery of oxygen-rich blood to the body's tissues. When the body's cells do not receive enough oxygen, they die. As the cells die, body tissue begins to suffer and die. As tissue begins to die, organs—such as the brain, heart, and kidneys—begin to fail. Death of the person eventually occurs if shock is not corrected. In fact, shock has been called "a momentary pause on the road to death."

Yet, shock—if recognized—proves a valuable ally to the health-care professional. Its early recognition may be the only sign of internal bleeding.

Causes of Shock

Shock, or poor tissue perfusion, can best be understood if you know what it takes for proper tissue oxygenation to occur. That is:

- *A properly functioning pump.* Heart attack, coronary artery disease, and cardiac tamponade (fluid leaking into the sac around the heart) all can contribute to a malfunction in the pumping action of the heart.

- *Enough oxygen-rich blood for the heart to pump.* Blood volume can decrease as a result of internal and external bleeding, fluid loss during prolonged illness or burns, and dehydration. (See Figure 3-8.)

- *Intact blood vessels through which blood can be pumped throughout the body.* When these "pipes," or vessels, are damaged, their ability to deliver oxygen-rich blood to cells is disrupted. Blood vessel failure also may be caused by extreme vessel dilation, which may occur with severe allergic reactions or spinal-cord injury.

What causes shock? An interruption of any of these three mechanisms—the pump (heart), fluid (blood), or pipes (arteries, veins, or capillaries).

🔔 FIRE DRILL

On the fireground, in order to "put the wet stuff on the red stuff," it is critical that the same three mechanisms be present. They are a functioning pump (centrifugal single or dual stage pump), a fluid to be pumped (water), and pipes or vessels (fire hose) to deliver the water to the fire. If any one of these three mechanisms is not working properly, we will not be able to extinguish the fire:

- Pump—if it fails, we cannot deliver water (blood) to the nozzle (cells).
- Fluid—if we run out of water (blood), no fluid will be available at the nozzle (cells).
- Pipes or vessels—if our hoseline breaks (arterial bleed), the amount of water (blood) delivered to the nozzle (cells) may be insufficient for extinguishment (proper oxygenation).

. . . And "shock" to the building—and its residents—will result!

Watch for shock in all trauma patients. They can lose fluids not only externally through hemorrhage, vomiting, or burns, but also internally through crush injuries and organ punctures.

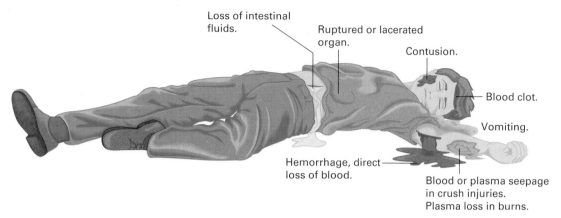

Loss of intestinal fluids.

Ruptured or lacerated organ.

Contusion.

Blood clot.

Vomiting.

Hemorrhage, direct loss of blood.

Blood or plasma seepage in crush injuries. Plasma loss in burns.

Figure 3-8   Loss of body fluids can be both external and internal.

Stages of Shock

Regardless of which component is malfunctioning —pump, blood, or blood vessels, shock (hypoperfusion) has three distinct phases. They are called *compensatory shock, decompensated shock,* and *irreversible shock* (Figures 3-9 and 3-10).

Compensatory Shock

In this first stage of shock, the body uses defense mechanisms to maintain normal function. They are so effective that an adult can lose up to 15% of total blood volume with little change in vital signs. If the condition does not get worse, the body will overcome it. Although subtle, the signs and symptoms of shock at this stage can be recognized:

◆ *Pale skin.* The vessels have constricted, forcing blood away from the skin into larger vessels lying further beneath the skin surface.

◆ *Slightly rapid heart rate.* With less blood, each blood cell must now make more trips through the body in order to deliver an adequate supply of oxygen to the cells.

◆ *Restlessness or anxiety.* The brain may not be receiving as much oxygen as it would like.

◆ *Blood pressure in the normal range.* With vessel constriction and increased heart rate, blood pressure will remain the same.

Decompensated Shock

At this stage, the body can no longer make up for reduced tissue perfusion of oxygenated blood.

> **FIRE DRILL**
>
> Waiting for blood pressure to drop in a bleeding patient is like waiting for the roof to collapse in a structure fire. If you wait, you probably won't be able to save the patient or the building!

Signs and symptoms are quite recognizable and include:

◆ *Extreme thirst,* which reflects the fluid deficit within the body.

◆ *Rapid, weak pulse.* It is rapid because the heart is beating faster than before in order to circulate what little fluid is in the vessels. It is weak because the vessels are now very narrow, and the volume moving through them is decreased.

◆ *Decreased blood pressure.* With little volume left and the vessels constricted as tight as they can be, pressure will begin to fall.

◆ *Cool and moist skin that is pale, gray, or mottled.* The body has now diverted all blood flow from the extremities and surface of the skin to the major organs.

◆ *Noticeable changes in the patient's mental status.* When oxygen delivery is compromised, the brain is the first organ to react.

When you perform an initial assessment, get an objective measurement of the patient's level of

Developing Shock

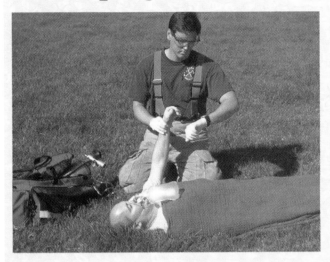

Figure 3-9a Compensatory shock: slight increase in pulse.

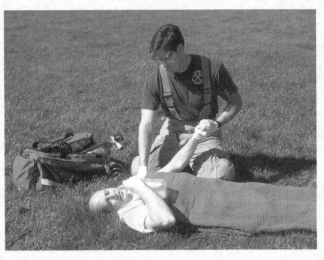

Figure 3-9b Compensatory shock: restlessness or anxiety.

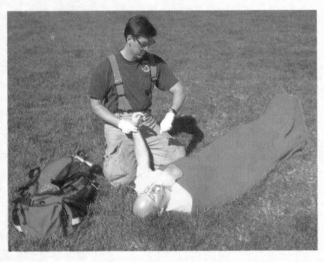

Figure 3-9c Decompensated shock: rapid, weak pulse.

responsiveness. For example, in addition to asking name, place, day, and date, have the patient repeat a certain number. You might say: "I'm giving you a number to repeat. It is the number 51. Can you say that number?" Throughout the assessment repeatedly ask "What is that number?" Note any changes in the patient's responses.

Irreversible Shock

Even with treatment, irreversible shock leads to death. At this stage, the blood vessels lose their

ability to constrict. This "relaxation" causes blood to pool away from vital organs. This leads to a dangerously low blood pressure, so low that entire organ systems begin to die.

◆ Emergency Care

It is vital for you to learn to see what is not obvious, but life threatening. Since trauma is a major cause of shock in patients, assume that any trauma patient is in compensatory shock until proven otherwise.

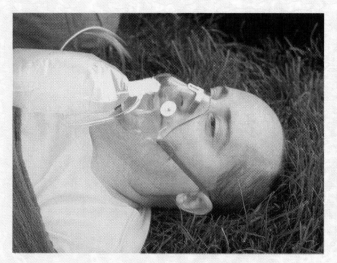

Figure 3-9d Decompensated shock: skin color changes and sweating.

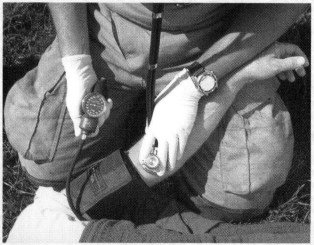

Figure 3-9e Decompensated shock: decreasing blood pressure.

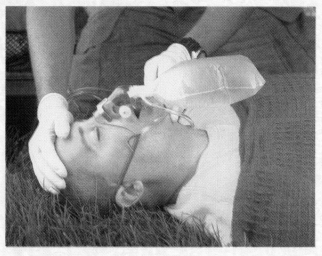

Figure 3-9f Decompensated shock: unresponsiveness.

Time is critical. Patients in shock (hypoperfusion) need to be transported quickly to an appropriate facility, such as a trauma center. In fact, the most important care you can provide is to identify the serious trauma patient and prepare him or her for transport as quickly as possible.

To provide emergency care, take BSI precautions and follow these steps (Figures 3-11 and 3-12):

1. **Maintain an open airway.** If breathing is adequate, administer high-flow oxygen with a nonrebreather mask at 15 liters per minute. Provide artificial ventilation, if necessary.

2. **Prevent further blood loss.** Since you cannot control internal bleeding, make sure you control all external bleeding. Use the DEPS principle.

3. **Elevate the lower extremities** about 8 to 12 inches (200 mm to 300 mm), if they are not injured. Also do not elevate if there are serious injuries to the head, neck, spine, chest, abdomen, or pelvis.

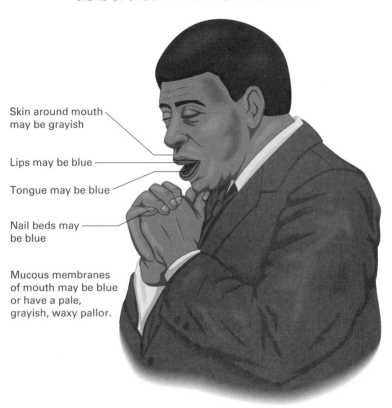

Skin around mouth
may be grayish

Lips may be blue

Tongue may be blue

Nail beds may
be blue

Mucous membranes
of mouth may be blue
or have a pale,
grayish, waxy pallor.

Figure 3-10   Signs of shock in a dark-skinned patient.

Figure 3-11   Administer oxygen to a patient in shock, if you are allowed to do so.

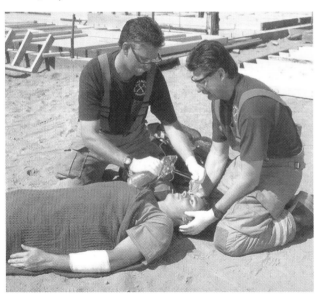

Figure 3-12   Elevate the lower extremities 8 to 12 inches (200 mm to 300 mm), if appropriate.

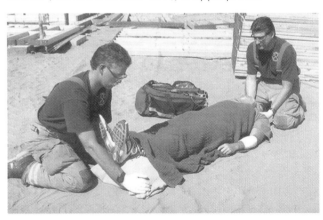

4. **Keep the patient warm.** But do not overheat. Use a blanket over and under the patient to help maintain a normal body temperature.

5. **Do not give the patient anything to eat or drink.** If the patient is experiencing nausea, eating or drinking may result in vomiting. The last thing you need is to create an airway problem!

6. **Provide emergency care for specific injuries.** But do so only if it will not delay transport.

Report your initial assessment findings to the transport crew as soon as possible. This will allow them to choose the appropriate response. They also may be able to initiate other EMS system resources available in your community (such as air transport, trauma center notification, and so on).

 ## ON SCENE FOLLOW-UP

At the beginning of this chapter, you read that fire service First Responders were providing emergency care to a patient who fell from a roof while removing holiday lights. To see how chapter information applies to this emergency, read the following. It describes how the call was completed.

ONGOING ASSESSMENT

I performed another assessment of Dan's vital signs. They were breathing 28, pulse 144, and blood pressure 128/70. I asked Dan if he would repeat the number I gave him and he said "Sure. The number is, ah, 51 . . . I think, right?"

PATIENT HAND-OFF

At this time, the ambulance crew had arrived. I gave the following report to Paramedic Bill Post:

"This is Dan Williams, a 41-year-old male who fell about 18 to 20 feet (6 m to 7 m) from this roof onto the lawn where he is lying. Upon arrival, Dan was alert and oriented. He responded appropriately to our questions, and stated that he fell face first. His wife confirms this. He denies any loss of consciousness. His chief complaint is abdominal pain. Our physical exam reveals left

upper quadrant tenderness, with some rigidity. Dan states he has no other medical conditions, is taking ibuprofen for arthritis of his knee, and has no allergies.

Baseline vital signs: BP was 130/70, pulse 120, breathing 28. He denies any shortness of breath. He would like something to drink. When we told him no, he became agitated. I also gave him the number 51 to repeat back to me, which he could do 10 minutes ago. However, he wasn't sure what the number was, when I asked him just as you arrived on scene. Also, his latest vitals are BP 128/70, pulse 144, breathing 28. We have taken spinal precautions and placed him on oxygen at 15 liters per minute with a nonrebreather mask. How else can we help you?"

If in the initial assessment you observe significant external bleeding or any signs of internal bleeding in your patient, treat the patient for shock immediately. However, remember that when the mechanism of injury suggests possible internal bleeding—even if you observe no signs or symptoms, treat the patient for shock until proven otherwise. Do not wait for signs of shock to develop.

Chapter Review

Severe bleeding is controlled during the initial assessment. Only airway and breathing care would take priority. Be assured, however, that even severe bleeding can be controlled by the simple methods described in this chapter: direct pressure, elevation, pressure points, and splinting. Experienced EMS personnel will tell you that these methods work. Use them appropriately and confidently.

FIRE COMPANY REVIEW

Page references where answers may be found or supported are provided at the end of each question.

Section 1

1. How would you describe the differences between arterial, venous, and capillary bleeding? (p. 52)

2. What four methods of controlling external bleeding are available for the fire service First Responder? (pp. 52, 54–56)

3. What are at least four signs and symptoms that the fire service First Responder may encounter in a patient suffering from internal bleeding? (pp. 57–58)

4. What is the emergency medical care of a patient with internal bleeding? (p. 58)

Section 2

5. What is the definition of the term "shock"? (p. 58)

6. What are the signs and symptoms of a patient suffering from shock? (pp. 59–60)

7. How should you provide emergency care for a patient in shock? (pp. 60–61, 63)

RESOURCES TO LEARN MORE

"Management of Shock" in Moore, E.E., et al., eds. *Trauma,* Second Edition. Norwalk, CT: Appleton-Lange, 1991.

EMERGENCY CARE OF EXTERNAL BLEEDING

Apply direct pressure to the wound with a gloved hand or sterile dressing.

Elevate the bleeding extremity.

If bleeding is not controlled, use the appropriate pressure point.

Once bleeding is controlled in an extremity, immobilize the limb by splinting in order to prevent reoccurrence, if necessary.

Glossary of Abbreviations

A

ABCs: airway, breathing, circulation.
ACLS: advanced cardiac life support.
ADA: Americans with Disabilities Act.
AED: automated external defibrillator.
AHA: American Heart Association.
AIDS: acquired immune deficiency syndrome.
ALS: advanced life support.
ATV: all-terrain vehicle.
AVPU: alert, verbal, painful, unresponsive.

B

BLS: basic life support.
BP: blood pressure.
BSA: body surface area.
BSI: body substance isolation.
BVM: bag-valve-mask device.

C

CDC: Centers for Disease Control.
CHEMTREC: Chemical Transportation Emergency Center.
CISD: critical incident stress debriefing.
CISM: critical incident stress management.
cm: centimeters.
COPD: chronic obstruction pulmonary disease.
CPR: cardiopulmonary resuscitation.
CVA: cerebral vascular accident.

D

DNR orders: do not resuscitate orders.
DOT: U.S. Department of Transportation.
DOTS: deformities, open injuries, tenderness, swelling.

E

EIR: emergency incident rehabilitation.
EKG: electrocardiogram.
EMD: emergency medical dispatcher.
EMS: emergency medical services.
EMT: emergency medical technician.

EMT-B: EMT-Basic.
EMT-I: EMT-Intermediate.
EMT-P: EMT-Paramedic.
EPA: Environmental Protection Agency.
ERT: emergency response team.
ETA: estimated time of arrival.

F

FBAO: foreign body airway obstruction.
FCC: Federal Communications Commission.
FGC: fire ground command.

H

hazmat: hazardous material.
HBIG: hepatitis B immunoglobulin.
HBV: hepatitis B virus.
HEPA respirator: high efficiency particulate air respirator.
Hg: mercury.
HIV: human immunodeficiency virus.

I

ICS: incident command system.
IFSTA: International Fire Service Training Association.
IMS: Incident Management System.
IV: intravenous.

L

L: liter.
LZ: landing zone.

M

m: meter.
MCI: multiple-casualty incident.
MCS: multiple-casualty situation.
ml: milliliters.
mm: millimeters.
MOI: mechanism of injury.
MSDS: material safety data sheets.

N

NFPA: National Fire Protection Association.
NHTSA: National Highway Traffic Safety Administration.
NIOSH: National Institute of Occupational Safety and Health.
NOI: nature of illness.
NREMT: National Registry of Emergency Medical Technicians.

O

O$_2$: oxygen.
OB kit: obstetrical kit.
OPQRRRST: onset, provocation, quality, region, radiation, relief, severity, time of pain.
OSHA: Occupational Safety and Health Administration.

P

PCR: prehospital care report.
PEA: pulseless electrical activity.

PMS-CR: pulse, movement, sensation, capillary refill.
PPE: personal protective equipment.
PSAP: public service answering point.
psi: pounds per square inch.

S

SAED: semi-automated external defibrillator.
SAMPLE: signs and symptoms, allergies, medications, pertinent medical history, last oral intake, events.
SCBA: self-contained breathing apparatus.
SIDS: sudden infant death syndrome.
SOP/G: standard operating procedure/guideline.
START system: simple triage and rapid treatment system.

T

TB: tuberculosis.
TIA: transient ischemic attack.

Glossary of Terms

abandonment: a legal term referring to discontinuing emergency medical care without making sure that another health-care professional with equal or better training has taken over.

abdominal cavity: the space below the diaphragm and continuous with the pelvic cavity.

abrasion: an open wound caused by scraping, rubbing, or shearing away of the epidermis.

abuse: improper or excessive action so as to injure or cause harm.

accessory muscles: additional muscles; in regard to breathing, these are the muscles of the neck and the muscles between the ribs.

activated charcoal: a finely ground charcoal that is very absorbent and is sometimes used as an antidote to some ingested poisons.

acute abdomen: a sharp, severe abdominal pain with rapid onset.

advance directive: a patient's instructions, written in advance, regarding the kind of resuscitation efforts that should be made in a life-threatening emergency.

afterbirth: the placenta after it separates from the uterine wall and delivers.

agonal respirations: reflex gasping with no regular pattern or depth; a sign of impending cardiac or respiratory arrest.

airway adjunct: an artificial airway.

alimentary tract: the food passageway that extends from the mouth to the anus.

altered mental status: a change in a patient's normal level of responsiveness.

alveoli: the air sacs of the lungs. *Singular* alveolus.

amniotic sac: a sac of fluid in which the fetus floats.

amputation: an injury that occurs when a body part is severed from the body.

anatomical position: a position in which the patient is standing erect with arms down at the sides, palms facing front.

aneurysm: an enlarged or burst artery.

antecubital space: the hollow, or front, of the elbow.

anterior: a term of direction or position meaning toward the front. *Opposite of* posterior.

aorta: major artery that starts at the left ventricle of the heart and carries oxygen-rich blood to the body.

apical pulse: an arterial pulse point located under the left breast.

arterial bleeding: recognized by bright red blood spurting from a wound.

arteries: blood vessels that take blood away from the heart.

arterioles: the smallest arteries.

artificial ventilation: a method of assisting breathing by forcing air into a patient's lungs.

asphyxia: suffocation.

aspirate: to inhale materials into the lungs.

assault: the threat of physical harm.

atria: the two upper chambers of the heart. *Singular* atrium.

auscultation: a method of examination that involves listening for signs of injury or illness.

autonomic nervous system: the part of the nervous system that handles involuntary activities.

avulsion: an open wound that is characterized by a torn flap of skin or soft tissue that is either still attached to the body or pulled off completely.

bag of waters: amniotic sac.

battery: unlawful physical contact.

behavior: the way a person acts or performs.

behavioral emergency: a situation in which a patient exhibits behavior that is unacceptable or intolerable to the patient, family, or community.

birth canal: a passage made of the cervix and vagina.

blanch: to lose color.

blood pressure: the amount of pressure the surging blood exerts against the arterial walls.

blood vessels: a closed system of tubes through which blood flows.

bloody show: the mucous plug that is discharged during labor.

blunt trauma: injuries caused by a sudden blow or force that has a crushing impact.

body armor: a garment made of a synthetic material that resists penetration by bullets.

body mechanics: the safest and most efficient methods of using the body to gain a mechanical advantage.

body substance isolation (BSI): a strict form of infection control based on the premise that all blood and body fluids are infectious.

brachial pulse point: an arterial pulse that can be felt on the inside of the arm between the elbow and the shoulder.

bracing: exerting an opposing force against two parts of a stable surface with your body; in EMS, usually refers to a safety precaution taken while riding in an ambulance patient compartment.

bronchi: the two main branches of the trachea, which lead to the lungs. *Singular* bronchus.

burn center: a medical facility devoted to treatment of burns, often including long-term care and rehabilitation.

burnout: a state of exhaustion and irritability caused by the chronic stress of work-related problems in an emotionally charged environment.

――――――― C ―――――――

capillaries: the smallest blood vessels through which the exchange of fluid, oxygen, and carbon dioxide takes place between the blood and tissue cells.

capillary bleeding: recognized by dark red blood that oozes slowly from a wound.

capillary refill: the time it takes for capillaries that have been compressed to refill with blood.

cardiac arrest: the sudden cessation of circulation.

cardiac muscle: one of three types of muscles; makes up the walls of the heart.

carotid pulse point: an arterial pulse that can be felt on either side of the neck.

catheter: a hollow tube that is part of a suctioning system. *Also called* tonsil tip *or* tonsil sucker.

central nervous system: the brain and the spinal cord.

cerebrospinal fluid: a water cushion that helps to protect the brain and spinal cord from trauma.

cervical spine: the neck, formed by the first seven vertebrae.

cervix: the neck of the uterus.

chain of survival: term used by the American Heart Association for a series of interventions that provide the best chance of survival for a cardiac-arrest patient.

chief complaint: the reason that EMS was called stated in the patient's own words.

child: according to AHA standards, any patient who is age one to eight years old.

chronic: of long duration.

circulatory system: the system that transports blood to all parts of the body.

clamping injury: a soft-tissue injury usually caused by a body part being stuck in an area smaller than itself.

clavicle: the collarbone.

cleaning: the process of washing a soiled object with soap and water. *See* disinfecting *and* sterilizing.

closed wound: an injury to the soft tissues beneath unbroken skin.

coccyx: the tail bone, formed by four fused vertebrae. *Also called* coccygeal spine.

colicky pain: cramps that occur in waves.

command: person responsible for the management of a multiple-casualty incident.

competent: in EMS a competent adult is one who is lucid and able to make an informed decision about medical care.

complete foreign body airway obstruction: all air exchange has stopped because an object fully occludes the patient's airway.

complex access: the process of gaining access to a patient which requires the use of tools and specialized equipment.

consent: permission to provide emergency care. *See* expressed consent *and* implied consent.

constrict: get smaller.

contusion: a bruise; a type of closed soft-tissue injury.

cornea: the anterior part of a transparent coating that covers the iris and pupil.

cranium: the bones that form the top (including the forehead), back, and sides of the skull.

crepitus: the sound or feeling of bones grinding against each other.

cribbing: a system of wood or other materials used to support an object.

cricoid cartilage: shaped like a ring, this is the lowermost cartilage of the larynx.

critical incident: any situation that causes a rescuer to experience unusually strong emotions which interfere with the ability to function either during the incident or later.

critical incident stress debriefing (CISD): a session usually held within three days of a critical incident in which a team of peer counselors and mental health professionals help rescuers work through the emotions that normally follow a critical incident.

cross-finger technique: a method of opening a patient's clenched jaw.

crowing: a sound made during respiration similar to the cawing of a crow, which may mean the muscles around the larynx are in spasm.

crowning: the appearance of the baby's head or other body part at the opening of the birth canal.

crushing injury: an open or closed injury to soft tissues and underlying organs that is the result of a sudden blow or a blunt force that has a crushing impact.

cyanosis: bluish discoloration of the skin and mucous membranes; a sign that body tissues are not receiving enough oxygen.

--- **D** ---

debriefing: a technique used to help rescuers work through their emotions within 24 to 72 hours after a critical incident.

deep: a term of position, meaning remote or far from the surface. *Opposite of* superficial.

defibrillation: the process by which an electrical current is sent to the heart to correct fatal heart rhythms.

defusing: a short, informal type of debriefing held within hours of a critical incident.

dermis: second layer of skin. *See* epidermis *and* subcutaneous tissue.

diabetes: a disease in which the normal relationship between glucose (sugar) and insulin is altered.

diaphragm: a muscle, located between the thoracic and abdominal cavities, that moves up and down during respiration.

diastolic pressure: the result of the relaxation of the heart between contractions. *See* systolic pressure.

dilate: enlarge.

direct medical control: refers to an EMS medical director or another physician giving orders to an EMS rescuer at the scene of an emergency

via telephone, radio, or in person. *See* indirect medical control.

disinfecting: the process of cleaning plus using a disinfectant, such as alcohol or bleach, to kill microorganisms on an object. *See* cleaning *and* sterilizing.

distal: a term of direction or position, meaning distant or far away from the point of reference, which is usually the torso. *Opposite of* proximal.

Do Not Resuscitate (DNR) orders: documents that relate the wish of the chronically or terminally ill patient not to be resuscitated. *See* advance directive.

dorsalis pedis pulse: an arterial pulse point that can be felt at the top of the foot on the great toe side.

dressing: a covering for a wound.

drowning: death from suffocation due to immersion in water.

drug abuse: self-administration of one or more drugs in a way that is not in accord with approved medical or social practice.

duty to act: the legal obligation to care for a patient who requires it.

dyspnea: shortness of breath.

--- **E** ---

ecchymosis: black and blue discoloration.

emancipated minor: a minor who is married, pregnant, a parent, in the armed forces, or financially independent and living away from home with permission of the courts.

embolus: a mass of undissolved matter in the blood. *Plural* emboli.

emergency medical services (EMS) system: a network of resources that provides emergency medical care to victims of sudden illness or injury.

emergency move: a move made when there is immediate danger to the patient, usually performed by a single rescuer.

EMT-Basic (EMT-B): an emergency medical technician trained to the level above the EMS First Responder.

EMT-Intermediate (EMT-I): an emergency medical technician trained to a higher level than the EMT-Basic and First Responder.

EMT-Paramedic (EMT-P): the most highly trained emergency medical technician in EMS.

enhanced 9-1-1: with this type of 9-1-1 service, the EMS dispatcher is able to see the street address and phone number of a caller on a computer screen.

epidermis: outermost layer of skin. *See* dermis *and* subcutaneous tissue.

epiglottis: a leaf-shaped structure that prevents foreign objects from entering the trachea during swallowing.

epiglottitis: a bacterial infection of the epiglottis.

esophagus: a passageway at the lower end of the pharynx that leads to the stomach.

evisceration: the protrusion of organs from an open wound.

expiration: breathing out; exhaling.

expressed consent: permission that must be obtained from every responsive, competent adult patient before emergency medical care may be rendered.

external: a term of position, meaning outside. *Opposite of* internal.

extremities: the limbs of the body.

extrude: to push or force out.

eye orbits: eye sockets; the bones in the skull that hold the eyeballs.

--- F ---

fallopian tube: the tube or duct that extends up from the uterus to a position near an ovary.

femoral pulse point: an arterial pulse that can be felt in the area of the groin in the crease between the abdomen and the thigh.

femur: the bone in the thigh, or upper leg.

fibula: one of the bones of the lower leg.

finger sweep: a technique used to remove a foreign object from the mouth.

First Responder: the first person on the scene with emergency medical care skills, typically trained to the most basic EMS level.

flail chest: a closed chest injury resulting in the chest wall becoming unstable.

flail segment: an area of chest wall between broken ribs that becomes free-floating.

fontanel: a soft spot lying between the cranial bones of the skull of an infant.

freelancing: uncoordinated or undirected activity at the emergency scene.

frostbite: freezing or near freezing of a specific body part. *Also called* local cold injury.

full thickness burn: a burn that extends through all layers of skin and may involve muscles, organs, and bone.

--- G ---

gastric distention: inflation of the stomach.

genitalia: reproductive organs.

globe: eyeball.

glucose: a type of sugar.

grieving process: the process by which people cope with death.

guarding position: a position in which the patient is on his or her side with knees drawn up toward the abdomen.

--- H ---

hand-off report: a report of the patient's condition and the care that was given, made to the EMS personnel who take over patient care.

hazardous material: a substance that in any quantity poses threat or unreasonable risk to life, health, or property if not properly controlled.

hazmat: hazardous material.

head-tilt/chin-lift maneuver: a manual technique used to open the airway of an uninjured patient. *See* jaw-thrust maneuver.

Heimlich maneuver: a technique used to dislodge and expel a foreign body airway obstruction. *Also called* subdiaphragmatic abdominal thrusts *and* abdominal thrusts.

hematoma: a collection of blood beneath the skin.

hemodilution: an increase in volume of blood plasma resulting in reduced concentration of red blood cells.

hemothorax: collapse of the lungs caused by bleeding in the chest.

humane restraints: padded soft leather or cloth straps used to tie a patient down in order to keep the patient from hurting him- or herself and others.

humerus: the bone that extends from the shoulder to the elbow.

hydration: the addition of water.

hyperthermia: fever or raised body temperature.

hyperventilation: rapid breathing common to diseases such as asthma and pulmonary edema; the syndrome is common to anxiety-induced states.

hypoglycemia: low blood sugar.

hypoperfusion: *See* shock.

hypothermia: the overall reduction of body temperature. *Also called* generalized cold emergency.

hypoxemia: a condition caused by a deficiency of oxygen in the blood.

hypoxia: decreased levels of oxygen in the blood.

————————— I —————————

ilium: one of the bones that form the pelvis. *Plural* ilia.

immobilize: to make immovable.

impaled object: an object that is embedded in an open wound.

implied consent: the assumption that in an emergency a patient who cannot give permission for emergency medical care would give it if he or she could.

incontinent: unable to retain.

index of suspicion: an informal measure of anticipation that certain types of mechanisms produce specific types of injury.

indirect medical control: refers to EMS system design, protocols and standing orders, education for EMS personnel, and quality management. *See* direct medical control.

infant: according to AHA standards, a patient from birth to one year old.

infectious disease: a disease that can spread from one person to another.

inferior: a term of direction or position, meaning toward or closer to the feet. *Opposite of* superior.

inferior vena cava: the great vein that collects blood from the lower body and delivers it to the heart.

initial assessment: part of patient assessment, conducted directly after the scene size-up, in which the rescuer identifies and treats life-threatening conditions.

inspection: method of examination that involves looking for signs of injury or illness.

inspiration: breathing in; inhaling.

insulin: a hormone secreted by the pancreas, essential to the metabolism of blood sugar.

intercostal: between the ribs.

internal: a term of position, meaning inside. *Opposite of* external.

internal bleeding: bleeding that occurs inside the body.

involuntary muscle: *See* smooth muscle.

ischium: the lower portion of the pelvis or hip bone. *Plural* ischia.

————————— J —————————

jaw-thrust maneuver: a manual technique used to open the airway of an unresponsive patient who is injured or any patient who has suspected spine injury. *See* head-tilt/chin-lift maneuver.

————————— K —————————

kinematics of trauma: the science of analyzing mechanisms of injury.

————————— L —————————

labor: the term used to describe the process of childbirth.

laceration: an open wound of varying depth.

larynx: the voice box.

lateral: a term of direction or position, meaning to the left or right of the midline. *See* medial.

lateral recumbent position: the patient is lying on the left or right side.

level of responsiveness: mental status, usually characterized as alert, verbal, responsive to pain, or unresponsive.

ligaments: tissues that connect bone to bone.

litter: portable stretcher or cot.

local cold injury: freezing or near freezing of a specific body part. *Also called* frostbite.

log roll: a method of turning a patient without causing injury to his or her spine.

lumbar spine: the lower back, formed by five vertebrae.

————————— M —————————

manual traction: applying a pulling force to a body part in order to align it.

mechanism of injury (MOI): the force or forces that cause an injury.

meconium staining: a greenish or brownish color to the amniotic fluid, which means the unborn infant had a bowel movement.

medial: a term of direction or position, meaning toward the midline or center of the body. *See* lateral.

medical director: in EMS this person is the physician legally responsible for the clinical and patient-care aspects of an EMS system.

medical identification tag: medallion or bracelet that identifies a specific medical condition such as an allergy, epilepsy, or diabetes.

medical patient: a patient who is ill, not injured.

minor: any person under the legally defined age of an adult; usually under the age of 18 or 21.

mouth-to-barrier device ventilation: a technique of artificial ventilation that involves the use of a barrier device such as a face shield to blow air into the mouth of a patient.

mouth-to-mask ventilation: a technique of artificial ventilation that involves the use of a pocket mask with one-way valve to blow air into the mouth of a patient.

mouth-to-mouth ventilation: a technique of artificial ventilation that involves blowing air directly from the rescuer's mouth into the mouth of a patient.

multiple-casualty incident (MCI): any emergency where three or more patients are involved.

musculoskeletal system: a system made up of the skeleton and muscles, which help to give the body shape, protect the organs, and provide for movement.

myocardial infarction: heart attack.

N
---

nasal airway: *See* nasopharyngeal airway.

nasal cannula: an oxygen delivery device characterized by two soft plastic tips, which are inserted a short distance into the nostrils.

nasopharyngeal airway: an artificial airway positioned in the nose and extending down to the larynx. *Also called* nasal airway.

nasopharynx: the nasal part of the pharynx.

nature of illness (NOI): the type of medical condition or complaint a patient may be suffering.

neglect: refers to giving insufficient attention or respect to someone who has a claim to that attention and respect.

negligence: the act of deviating from the accepted standard of care through carelessness, inattention, disregard, inadvertence, or oversight that was accidental but avoidable.

nervous system: the body system that controls the voluntary and involuntary activity of the body; includes the brain, spinal cord, and nerves.

non-accidental trauma: injuries such as those caused by child abuse.

non-emergency move: a move made by several rescuers usually after a patient has been stabilized. *Also called* non-urgent move.

nonrebreather mask: an oxygen delivery device characterized by an oxygen reservoir bag and a one-way valve.

O
---

occlude: to block, close up, or obstruct.

occlusive dressing: a dressing that can form an air-tight and sometimes water-tight seal.

open injury: an injury to the soft tissues that is caused by a blow and results in breaking the skin.

oral airway: *See* oropharyngeal airway.

orbit: eye socket; the bones in the skull that hold the eyeball.

oropharyngeal airway: an artificial airway positioned in the mouth and extending down to the larynx. *Also called* oral airway.

oropharynx: the central part of the pharynx.

overdose: an emergency that involves poisoning by drugs or alcohol.

P
---

packaging: refers to getting the patient ready to be moved and includes procedures such as stabilizing impaled objects and immobilizing injured limbs.

palmar surface method: a method used to estimate the percent of body surface area involved in a burn injury.

palpation: method of examination that involves feeling for signs of injury or illness.

palpitations: a sensation of abnormal rapid throbbing or fluttering of the heart

paradoxical breathing: a segment of the chest moves in the opposite direction to the rest of the chest during respiration; typically seen with a flail segment.

paramedic: *See* EMT-Paramedic.

parietal pleura: the membrane that covers the internal chest wall.

partial foreign body airway obstruction: refers to an object that is caught in the throat but does not totally occlude the airway and prevent breathing.

partial thickness burn: a burn that involves both the epidermis and dermis.

patella: the knee cap.

patent airway: an airway that is open and clear of obstructions.

pathogens: microorganisms such as bacteria and viruses, which cause disease.

patient history: facts about the patient's medical history that are relevant to the patient's condition.

pediatric center: medical facility devoted to the treatment of infants and children.

pediatric patients: patients who are infants or children.

pelvic cavity: a space bound by the lower part of the spine, the hip bones, and the pubis.

pelvis: the hips.

penetration/puncture wound: an open wound that is the result of a sharp, pointed object being pushed or driven into soft tissues.

perfusion: refers to the circulation of blood throughout a body organ or structure.

perinatal center: medical facility devoted to the treatment of high-risk pregnant patients.

peripheral nervous system: the portion of the nervous system that is located outside the brain and spinal cord; the nerves.

personal protective equipment (PPE): equipment used by a rescuer to protect against injury and the spread of infectious disease.

pharynx: the throat.

placenta: a disk-shaped inner lining of the uterus that provides nourishment and oxygen to a fetus.

pleura: the membranes that enfold both lungs.

pleural cavity: the space between the visceral pleura and the parietal pleura.

pneumothorax: collapse of the lungs caused by air in the chest.

poison center: medical facility devoted to providing information for treatment of poisoning victims.

posterior: a term of direction or position, meaning toward the back. *Opposite of* anterior.

posterior tibial pulse: an arterial pulse point that can be felt behind the medial ankle bone.

potential crime scene: any scene that may require police support.

power grip: a technique used to get maximum force from hands while lifting and moving.

power lift: a technique used for lifting, especially helpful to rescuers with weak knees or thighs.

prehospital care: emergency medical treatment in the field before transport to a medical facility. *Also called* out-of-hospital care.

priapism: a constant erection of the penis.

prone: a position in which a patient is lying face down on his or her stomach. *Opposite of* supine.

protocols: written orders issued by the medical director that may be applied to patient care; a type of standing order.

proximal: a term of direction or position, meaning close or near the point of reference, which is usually the torso. *Opposite of* distal.

pubis: bone of the groin; the anterior portion of the pelvis.

public safety answering point (PSAP): location at which 9-1-1 calls are received.

pulmonary: concerning or involving the lungs.

pulmonary vein: vessel carrying oxygen-rich blood from the lungs to the left atrium of the heart.

pulse pressure: the difference between systolic blood pressure and diastolic blood pressure.

pulse: the wave of blood propelled through the arteries as a result of the pumping action of the heart.

pustules: raised areas of the skin that are filled with pus.

——————————— R ———————————

radial pulse point: an arterial pulse that can be felt on the palm side of the wrist.

radius: one of the bones of the forearm.

rape: sexual intercourse that is performed without consent and by compulsion through force, threat, or fraud.

rape trauma syndrome: a reaction to rape that involves four general stages: acute (impact) reaction, outward adjustment, depression, and acceptance and resolution.

rappelling: a special technique of getting down a cliff by means of a secured rope.

reasonable force: the minimum amount of force needed to keep a patient from injuring him- or herself and others.

recovery position: lateral recumbent position; used to allow fluids to drain from the patient's mouth instead of into the airway.

referred pain: pain felt in a part of the body that is different from its actual point of origin.

rehydration: replacement of water and electrolytes lost in sweating.

relative skin temperature: an assessment of skin temperature obtained by touching the patient's skin.

respiration: the passage of air into and out of the lungs.

respiratory arrest: the cessation of spontaneous breathing.

respiratory distress: shortness of breath or a feeling of air hunger with labored breathing.

respiratory system: organs involved in the interchange of gases between the body and the environment.

responsive: conscious; acting or moving in response to stimulus.

retraction: a pulling inward.

rule of nines: a method used to estimate the percent of body surface area involved in a burn injury.

——————— S ———————

sacrum: the lower part of the spine, formed by five fused vertebrae.

scapulae: the shoulder blades. *Singular* scapula.

scene size-up: an overall assessment of the emergency scene.

scope of care: actions and care legally allowed to be provided by a First Responder.

sector supervisor: at a multiple-casualty incident, the person in charge of overseeing a specific function such as transportation or rehab.

seizure: a sudden and temporary change in mental status caused by massive electrical discharge in the brain.

septum: a wall that divides two cavities.

sexual assault: any touch that the victim did not initiate or agree to and that is imposed by coercion, threat, deception, or threats of physical violence.

shock: a life-threatening, progressive condition that results from the inadequate delivery of oxygenated blood throughout the body.

shoulder girdle: consists of the clavicles and scapulae.

sign: any injury or medical condition that can be observed in a patient.

simple access: the process of gaining access to a patient without the use of tools.

skeletal muscle: one of three types of muscles; makes possible all deliberate acts such as walking and chewing. *Also called* voluntary muscle.

skull: a bony structure that houses and protects the brain.

smooth muscle: one of three types of muscles; found in the walls of tubelike organs, ducts, and blood vessels. *Also called* involuntary muscle.

sniffing position: position of a patient's head when the neck is flexed and the head is extended.

soft-tissue injuries: injuries to the skin, muscles, nerve, and blood vessels.

sphygmomanometer: instrument used to measure blood pressure. *Also called* blood pressure cuff.

spinal column: the column of bones, or vertebrae, that houses and protects the spinal cord.

spinal precautions: methods used to protect the spine from further injury; for First Responders, usually refers to the manual stabilization of the patient's head and neck until the patient is completely immobilized.

splint: a device used to immobilize a body part.

spontaneous abortion: miscarriage, or the loss of pregnancy before the twentieth week.

stabilize: to hold firmly and steadily.

standard of care: the care that would be expected to be provided to the same patient under the same circumstances by another First Responder who had received the same training.

standing orders: advance orders, rules, regulations, or step-by-step procedures to be taken under certain conditions; a type of indirect medical control.

status epilepticus: a seizure lasting longer than 10 minutes or seizures that occur consecutively without a period of responsiveness between them.

sterile: free of all microorganisms and spores.

sterilizing: process in which a chemical or other substance, such as superheated steam, is used to kill all microorganisms on an object. *See* cleaning *and* disinfecting.

sternum: breastbone.

stethoscope: instrument that aids in auscultating (listening) for sounds within the body.

stoma: a permanent surgically created opening that connects the trachea directly to the front of the neck.

stress: any change in the body's internal balance; occurs when external demands become greater than personal resources.

stridor: harsh, high-pitched sound made during inhalation, which may mean the larynx is swollen and blocking the upper airway.

stroke: loss of brain function caused by a blocked or ruptured blood vessel in the brain.

subcutaneous tissue: layer of fat beneath the skin.

sucking chest wound: open wound to the chest or back that bubbles or makes a sucking noise.

suctioning: using negative pressure created by a commercial device to keep the patient's airway clear.

superficial: term of position, meaning near the surface. *Opposite of* deep.

superficial burn: a burn that involves only the epidermis.

superior: a term of direction or position, meaning toward or closer to the head. *Opposite of* inferior.

supine: a position in which a patient is lying face up on his or her back. *Opposite of* prone.

symphysis pubis: the junction of the pubic bones on the midline in front; the bony eminence under the pubic hair.

symptom: any injury or medical condition that can only be described by the patient.

syrup of ipecac: a drug used to induce vomiting, usually in a patient who has ingested poison.

systolic pressure: the result of a contraction of the heart, which forces blood through the arteries. *See* diastolic pressure.

----------------- T -----------------

tendons: tissues that connect muscle to bone.

tension pneumothorax: a condition that is the result of an open chest wound, in which a severe build-up of air compresses the lungs and heart toward the uninjured side of the chest.

thoracic cavity: the space above the diaphragm and within the walls of the thorax. *Also called* chest cavity.

thoracic spine: the upper back, formed by 12 vertebrae.

thorax: the chest. *Also called* rib cage.

thrombus: a blood clot that obstructs a blood vessel.

tibia: one of the bones of the lower leg.

tongue-jaw lift: a technique used to draw the tongue away from the back of the throat and away from a foreign body that may be lodged there.

tourniquet: a constricting band used as a last resort on an extremity to apply pressure over an artery in order to control bleeding.

trachea: windpipe.

trauma center: a medical facility devoted to the treatment of injuries.

trauma patient: a patient who is injured.

triage: the process of sorting patients to determine the order in which they will receive care.

trimester: a three-month period.

tripod position: a position in which the patient is sitting upright, leaning forward, fighting to breathe.

----------------- U -----------------

ulna: one of the bones of the forearm.

umbilical cord: an extension of the placenta through which the fetus receives nourishment while in the uterus.

universal number: a phone number—usually 9-1-1— used in many areas to access emergency services including police, fire, rescue, and ambulance.

universal precautions: a form of infection control used against diseases spread by way of blood. *Also* BSI precautions.

unresponsive: unconscious; not acting or moving in response to stimulus.

uterus: the organ that contains the developing fetus.

----------------- V -----------------

veins: blood vessels that carry blood back to the heart from the rest of the body.

velocity: the speed at which an object moves.

venous bleeding: recognized by dark red blood that flows steadily from a wound.

ventilation: a method of assisting breathing by forcing air into a patient's lungs.

ventricles: the two lower chambers of the heart.

venules: the smallest kind of veins.

vertebrae: the 33 bone segments of the spinal column. *Singular* vertebra.

vesicles: small blisters or cysts that contain moisture.

visceral pleura: the membrane that covers the outer surface of the lungs.

vital signs: signs of life; assessments related to breathing, pulse, skin, pupils, and blood pressure.

voluntary muscle: *See* skeletal muscle.

—————— W ——————

wheals: itchy, raised, round marks on the skin that are red around the edges and white at the center.

withdrawal: a syndrome that occurs after a period of abstinence from the drugs or alcohol to which a person's body has become accustomed.

wound: a soft-tissue injury.

—————— X ——————

xiphoid process: the lowest portion of the sternum.